YOGA FOR
PREGNANCY

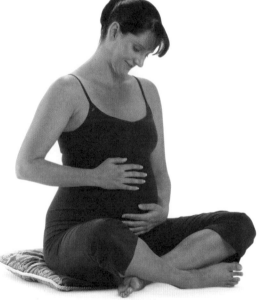

YOGA FOR PREGNANCY

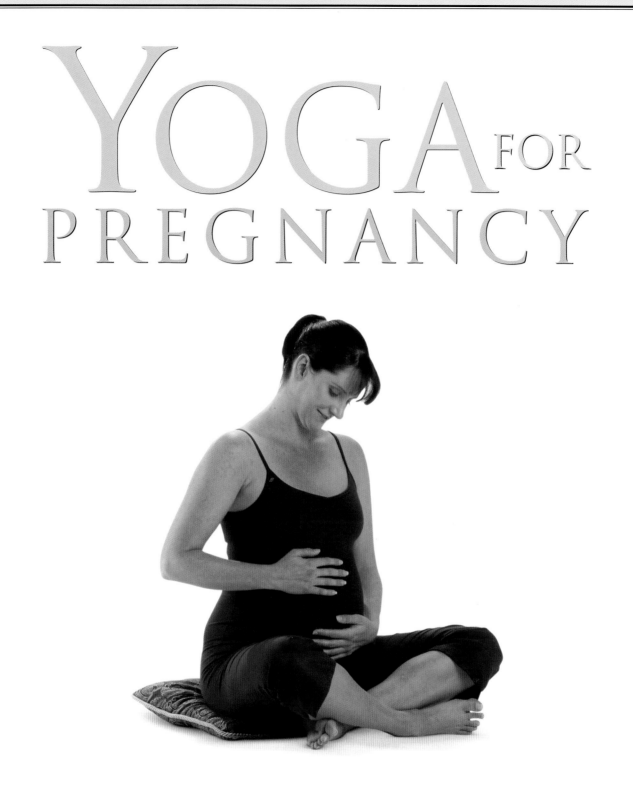

THERESA JAMIESON

HINKLER
BOOKS

Coordinator: Karen Moores
Editor: Margaret Barca
Graphic Artist: Andrew Cunningham
Photographer: UB Photo
Special thanks to Lisa Newland (37 weeks pregnant)

First published in 2004 by Hinkler Books Pty Ltd
17-23 Redwood Drive
Dingley, VIC 3172 Australia
www.hinklerbooks.com

Text © Theresa Jamieson 2004
Design © Hinkler Books Pty Ltd 2004

Printed and bound in China

ISBN 1 7412 1634 6

When practising *Yoga for Pregnancy*, always do the warm-up exercises
before attempting any individual postures.
It is recommended that you check with your doctor or health care
professional before commencing any exercise regime.
Whilst every care has been taken in the preparation of this material, the
Publishers and their respective employees or agents will not accept
responsibility for injury or damage occasioned to any person as a result of
participation in the activities described in this book.

CONTENTS

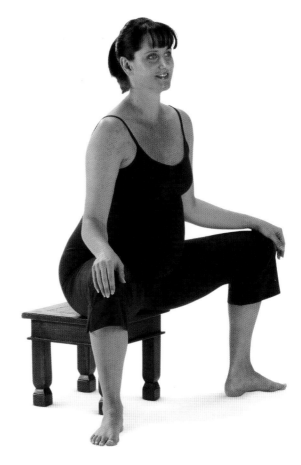

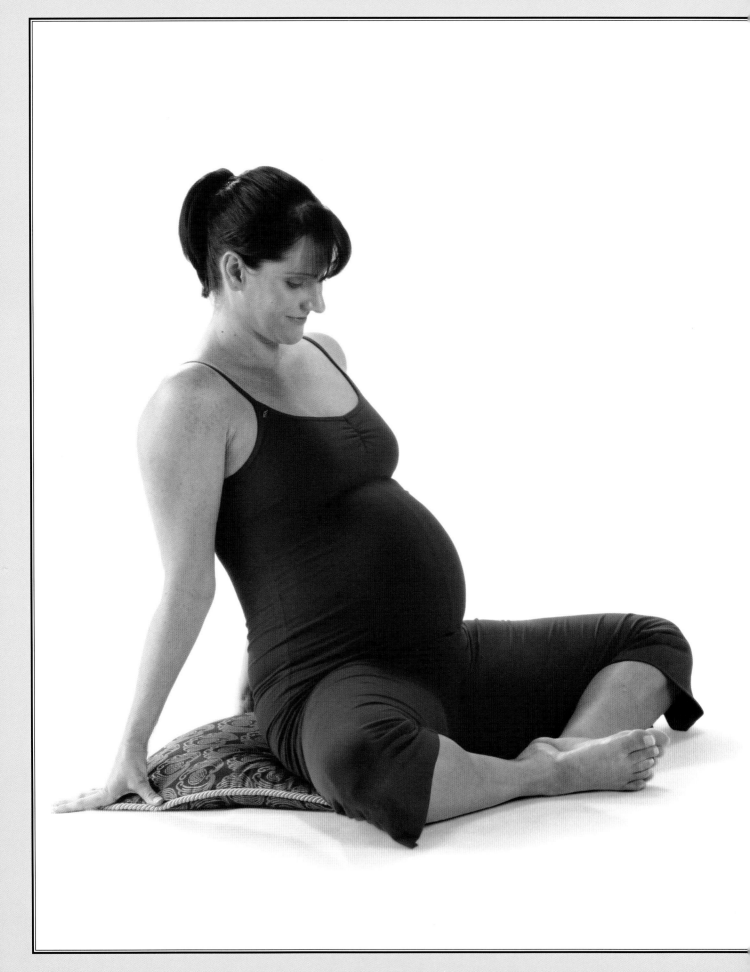

INTRODUCTION

The word yoga is derived from Sanskrit, the classical Indian language, and means union, or a coming together. The practice of yoga is a coming together of the mind, the body and the spirit.

The earliest writings on yoga are to be found in the Vedas, which date back 10,000 years and are considered to be amongst the most sacred texts of Hindu literature. It is from these ancient writings that the great Indian sage Patanjali constructed the Eight Fold Path of yoga, which is closely followed today by all yoga practitioners, either in its entirety or in the less conventional form that has made yoga so popular.

Patanjali's Eight Fold Path consists of:
1. *Yama* – self restraint
2. *Niyama* – self observation
3. *Asana* – physical postures
4. *Pranayama* – yoga breathing exercises
5. *Pratyahara* – mindfulness and withdrawal from the world
6. *Dharana* – concentration
7. *Dhyana* – meditation
8. *Samadi* – pure consciousness awareness.

Traditionally yoga includes many aspects, some of these involving years of teaching and dedication. However, today's yoga classes generally incorporate the most well-practised forms of yoga, being the postures (*asanas*), the breathing exercise (*pranayama*), concentration (*dharana*), and meditation (*dhyana*) as well as deep relaxation (*yoga nidra*). When they are used together in a yoga program they provide an extremely effective way of bringing about balance – physically, mentally and emotionally.

The different styles of yoga that are taught really depend on the teacher's personal approach, but generally all yoga covers the same principles and practices. The main difference is that some yoga is very gentle and more passive, with the emphasis on gentle stretching, breathing exercises and meditation, while other types of yoga are quite dynamic, strenuous and more physically demanding.

YOGA FOR PREGNANCY

Although yoga for pregnancy follows the same principals as all yoga, it is quite different from regular yoga because it is designed with the specific requirements of the pregnant woman and her ever-changing needs foremost in mind. Because of this, yoga for pregnancy is always safe, gentle and nurturing.

Pregnancy is a brief and precious time in your life where, like your baby in your womb, you are moving through a transformational phase of body and mind as you prepare to become a mother. It is a time filled with physical and emotional challenges as your body changes almost daily and your emotions shift as the hormonal levels adjust to the rapid changes of pregnancy. Yoga for pregnancy is possibly the most nurturing and gentle form of yoga, which benefits you in subtle, yet profound ways. It provides an ideal way to nurture and honour yourself during this transient and unique time.

PRECAUTIONS

Before you begin practising yoga during your pregnancy, it is essential that you consult with your doctor or midwife to confirm if there are any reasons why you should either take extra care during this time, or if it might not be appropriate to commence yoga at all. The safety and wellbeing of you and your baby are the most important considerations. Once you have the all clear, you can begin practising the yoga program detailed in this book and DVD with confidence and freedom from worry.

Yoga for pregnancy should always be gentle, relaxed and peaceful with the emphasis on it being safe and enjoyable, without straining or experiencing discomfort of any kind when doing a posture. You should not feel pain, either while practising yoga or after a session.

Generally it is recommended that you do not begin practising the yoga postures until after the first trimester, or around 12 to 14 weeks of pregnancy. However, the yoga breathing exercises, meditation and deep relaxation can be started as soon as you are aware of your pregnancy. Once you are in the second trimester the yoga exercises and postures can be commenced and these can be continued until full term pregnancy, as long as you feel well and are still enjoying your yoga.

When doing yoga during pregnancy remember that your body is constantly changing and therefore your needs will also change and in some cases you might have to make modifications and adjustments to your yoga program to continue in comfort and safety. When yoga is approached in this way it is always gentle and relaxing for the mind and the body. Importantly, you are taking the responsibility to practise within your own limitations and according to your own levels of fitness and flexibility. How far you are able to move into a pose or how flexible you are is irrelevant. The emphasis is on feeling as relaxed and comfortable as possible when you are holding the pose, aware that each breath helps you to move more fully into a position.

It is important to experience only a light stretch while practising yoga during this time, never straining or pushing beyond what is comfortable. There will be some exercises that you will do easily, while in other postures you will find your level of flexibility is quite limited. If you find a particular posture causes discomfort after your yoga time, discontinue this exercise and where possible seek advice from an experienced teacher who can explain a modified variation.

If you have high or low blood pressure, or have days where you are feeling faint or light-headed, avoid any of the postures where the head is down and follow the modifications recommended throughout the book and audio-visual.

Lower-back problems are one of the most common complaints during pregnancy and most of the postures recommended are an excellent and effective way to gain relief from these problems, or at the least to help prevent them becoming worse as the pregnancy progresses. However, some situations may require a complete cessation of a particular posture. Listen carefully to your body and take your time doing yoga.

If you have varicose veins or swollen feet, the full squatting pose is not recommended. Instead, practise this position on a stool or sitting on a step to relieve pressure on the legs and the feet. However, any of the squatting exercises that are not stationary and have continuous movement are not likely to cause a problem.

LYING ON YOUR BACK

From as early as 20 weeks many women feel very uncomfortable lying on their back due to the pressure the abdomen places on the vena cava, a major artery on the right side of the body. Although it isn't considered dangerous to spend time on your back, it can prove to be very uncomfortable and it is recommended you rest or sleep on your side instead. However, if you are experiencing discomfort but still wish to proceed with the spinal twists that are recommended lying on the back, begin by bending the knees and placing a cushion or folded towel under the right hip. This takes the weight away from the right side of the body and in many cases relieves the discomfort enough to complete the posture. If the problem persists always discontinue and practise the seated spinal twists instead as they have similar benefits.

This is also valuable knowledge to have if you are required to rest on your back for a medical procedure, such as an ultrasound, where it is necessary to be in this position for some time. Resting with the knees bent and a cushion placed under the right hip prevents backache and an unpleasant nausea that often accompanies lying on your back for a long time.

There might be days during your pregnancy when you are feeling exhausted or just a bit off-colour. In this case, rather than pushing yourself to do the yoga exercises, you would benefit far more from spending time in deep relaxation, meditation or practising the yoga breathing exercises. These will help to restore your energy levels and create a sense of wellbeing, mental and physical. In the unlikely event that bleeding occurs you must stop practising yoga immediately and seek medical advice.

Finally, if you also wish to attend yoga classes during your pregnancy always seek the expertise of a knowledgeable yoga teacher who specialises in this particular form of yoga and understands the varying needs of the pregnant woman.

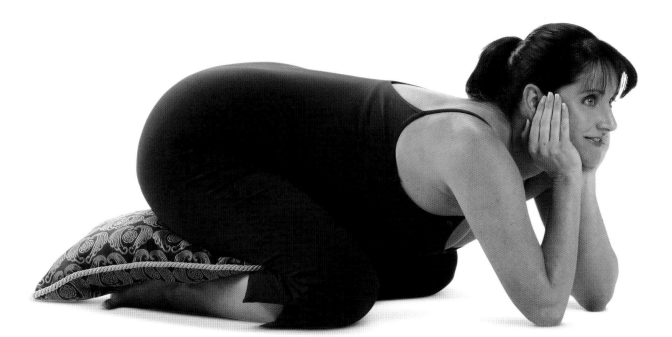

BENEFITS

There are many wonderful benefits to be gained from practising yoga during your pregnancy, benefits that you will feel almost immediately, even if you are new to yoga or are unable to begin practising until well into your pregnancy. The yoga postures that are recommended are specifically designed to gradually improve flexibility and suppleness whilst at the same time increasing general tone to the parts of the body that are most involved with pregnancy. These gentle exercises will also provide you with greater strength and stamina in preparation for labour and childbirth, and will help you to adjust more easily to the changes that naturally occur during this time.

Yoga benefits the whole person – physically, mentally and emotionally. With regular practice a sense of physical wellbeing and increased energy will be noticed, while emotional balance and stability will gradually improve, so that you can approach each day with a more calm and relaxed attitude.

The yoga breathing exercises, meditation and relaxation techniques will gently support and nourish you during this time and are excellent ways to gain relief from the stresses of modern living as well as the extra physical and emotional demands that are often felt during pregnancy.

While the different yoga practices are a wonderful way to maintain wellbeing during pregnancy, they will also help you to stay relaxed and calm when you are at home with your baby and moving into your new role as a mother. During those early days after the birth, the many benefits of these skills will enable you to enjoy these precious moments with your new baby, while these skills are also there for you to use for the rest of your life.

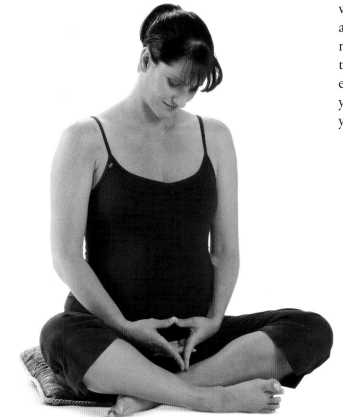

REQUIREMENTS

To enjoy yoga at home very little is required and most of what you will need, you probably already have. It is best to wear loose comfortable pants or shorts that are not restricting around the waist and pelvic region and a loose top. Shoes are not necessary for practising yoga. Two or three firm cushions will provide extra support and comfort and are necessary for modifying some of the seated positions. If the floor is too hard or cold a yoga mat is the ideal choice.

A bean bag is perfect for relaxation and meditation or when practising the yoga breathing exercises, especially if you are experiencing lower back pain or find sitting in a more traditional crossed-leg pose too uncomfortable. A small stool is useful when practising the squatting postures or when you are required to lean forward, especially if you find it difficult to do these exercises in comfort or if you have knee problems or suffer from high or low blood pressure. However, if you don't have a stool, sitting on a low step or resting with your hands on a step will provide the same support.

Always drink plenty of fluids especially in the warmer months. If you are still experiencing pregnancy sickness or are inclined to be hypoglycaemic, where the blood sugar levels drop mid morning and afternoon, it is quite acceptable to snack on a little light food to help overcome the discomfort.

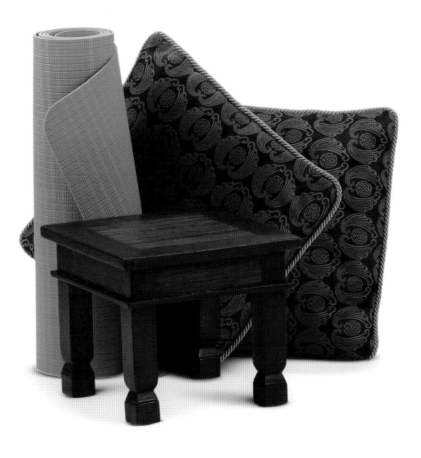

YOGA BREATHING

Essentially the breath is the foundation stone of all yoga practices, as every aspect of yoga centres around breathing and its natural rhythm and constancy. When the breath is followed by a quiet awareness, you become one with it as it moves gently and naturally through the body. From this pivotal point of breath awareness you become mindful of your body and begin to observe the atmosphere of your conscious mind and the nature of your thoughts.

Breath is the source of life. Throughout your life it is constantly with you, from the moment you take your first breath at birth until the final breath leaves your body and you die. Every breath is precious and has within it the gift of life, providing you with life-sustaining oxygen, without which you cannot exist. Awareness of this and the potential that each breath carries can be a potent meditation as it acknowledges that every moment you are alive and every breath that you take is truly a sacred one.

The yoga breathing practices are called *pranayama*. Translated from ancient sanskrit *prana* means energy or life-force, and *yama* means to control. When you develop a deeper understanding of *pranayama* you learn how to control your breathing more effectively and to utilise the *prana* or energy contained within every breath, and ultimately to live more fully and with increased awareness.

In many ways the practice of *pranayama* is even more important than the yoga postures, as breath awareness enables you to move through the postures and relax more fully into them. When yoga is practised without conscious breathing the benefits are far less and it cannot be called yoga in its purest form. By having a better understanding of the yoga breathing all areas of your life will be enriched and empowered, not only if you are pregnant but to all those who endeavour to understand and practise *pranayama*.

DEEP YOGA BREATHING

When deep yoga breathing is done correctly it flows slowly and rhythmically in and out of the body. The lungs, the diaphragm and the muscles of the chest and the upper back move in unison, resulting in a complete breath that is controlled yet at the same time relaxed. Deep yoga breathing is traditionally practised breathing in and out of the nose and is divided into abdominal breathing and thoracic breathing. The purpose of breathing deeply in this way is to utilise and absorb the available oxygen within each breath, ensuring optimum uptake of oxygen by the bloodstream to nourish the body, to fully cleanse the lungs and release the carbon dioxide when breathing out.

During times of stress where feelings of anger, anxiety and fear are present the breath usually becomes much more shallow and erratic, resulting in a depleted supply of available oxygen circulating in the bloodstream. When this continues for too long it eventually leads to unclear thinking and confusion. Correct breathing, however, ensures that optimum uptake of oxygen will be carried in the blood and throughout the whole body including the brain, resulting in clearer thinking and a break in the stress cycle. Sometimes a few deep breaths taken consciously at times of stress will not only delay the forthcoming emotions but will also give you the opportunity to think more clearly and therefore to act more calmly and rationally.

To increase awareness of the natural breath, place one hand over the abdomen and the other hand at the centre of the chest and feel the movement of the natural breath as it gently flows in and out of the body. This will help you to become more conscious of your breathing. It is also an excellent and reliable way to centre the mind and become more aware of your thoughts. The foundation of many meditation practices is based on witnessing the flow of the resting breath as it moves freely through the body. When practised even for a short time an increased sense of calmness and mindfulness will be experienced and enjoyed.

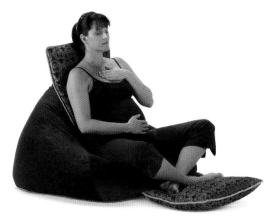

Abdominal breathing Place the hands on the abdomen with the fingertips touching at the navel centre. Imagine there is a balloon in the abdomen which inflates as you breathe in and deflates as you breathe out, noticing the fingertips moving apart slightly as you inhale and coming together again as you exhale. This is a slow, even, relaxed movement. When done correctly the diaphragm at the base of the lungs will flatten and lower, allowing the base of the lungs to fill for efficient breathing. Most people contract the abdomen inwards when they breathe in, which means they never breathe into the base of the lungs or utilise their full lung capacity.

Thoracic breathing Now place the hands at the centre of the chest with the fingertips touching and concentrate on feeling the breath moving deeply into the upper part of the body. As with abdominal breathing, the fingertips will come apart as the lungs expand and come together again as they contract.

Full yoga breathing To complete a full yoga breath concentrate on the breath moving deeply into the abdomen and then continue to breathe into the chest where you will feel a complete expansion of the lungs. As you breathe out the chest and the abdomen will relax and contract as the lungs are emptied. Breathe in and out evenly so that the inhalation is equal to the exhalation and the breath moves in a lovely, even rhythm. If you are feeling

NOTE

There are a number of other specific yoga breathing practices that are an invaluable part of any yoga program and are an important aspect of yoga for pregnancy; however these are too detailed to be discussed here.

breathless or light-headed after the deep breathing it is because you are not breathing evenly and are forcing the breath, making it become rigid and static, rather than allowing it to move freely through the body.

The full yoga breathing can be repeated 3 times to begin with. To perfect your breathing, repeat this three times each day. With regular practice you will have more control of how you breath and will be able to breathe much more slowly and deeply.

As a variation to the full yoga breathing, exhale through the mouth for a deep cleansing breath. This is an effective way to consciously relax the body and mind and to release tension.

Standing Poses

Arm Exercises with Deep Breathing

Benefits *This exercise encourages deep breathing with a full expansion of the lungs and a lovely stretch through the sides of the body.*

1 Stand with the feet a little apart and the arms relaxed beside the body. Breathe in deeply through the nose while raising the arms to the side. Complete the inhalation with the arms above the head.

2 Hold the breath for a short time, reaching up with the arms to feel a deep stretch through the sides of the body. The shoulders remain relaxed.

3 Breathe out through the nose as you lower the arms and relax. As an alternative you can breathe out through the mouth.

4 Repeat this exercise 3 times.

Note
Before commencing any postures practised from a standing position make sure that the shoulders are relaxed and the pelvis is tilted slightly forward to prevent a false arch developing in the lower back, as this can contribute to lower back discomfort and incorrect posture.

CHEST EXPANSION POSE

HASTA UTTHANASANA

Benefits *This valuable posture will help to release tension and tightness from the chest and the upper back and encourage better posture and more efficient breathing.*

1 Stand with the body relaxed, the feet a little apart and the hands crossed in front of the body. Slowly raise the arms in front of the body and stretch with the arms above the head.

2 Hold this stretch before slowly taking the arms back a little where the chest is opened and the shoulder blades come closer together, stretching the fingers wide for a full stretch.

3 Continue to lower the arms and relax. This can be repeated 3 times.

This exercise is practised very slowly and is not meant to be done in conjunction with the breathing. As a guideline, take 2 breaths as you raise the arms and 2 more as you lower them.

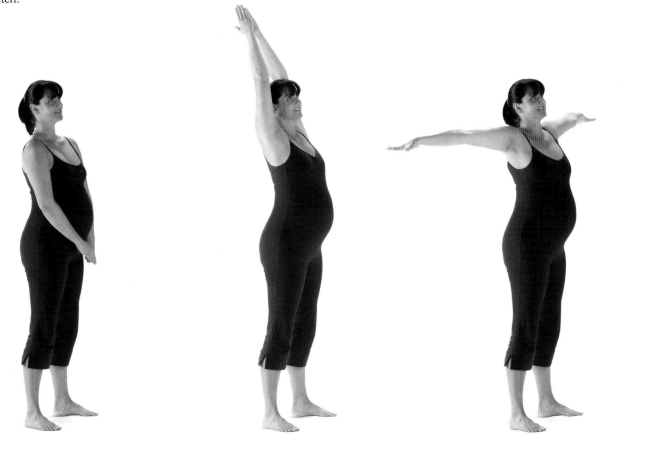

HEAD & NECK EXERCISES

GARDHANASANA

Benefits *Tension and tightness are relieved in the muscles of the neck, the upper back and the shoulders to give greater freedom of movement and improved flexibility. Allow the weight of the head to help you gradually ease into the stretch rather than forcing the head into the positions. If discomfort is felt, ease out of the stretch slightly until it feels comfortable and you are able to relax. Note that a full head rotation is not recommended.*

FORWARD AND BACK

1 Stand with the body relaxed and the feet a little apart, the arms loose beside the body.

2 Lower the head towards the chest and hold this position for 2 or 3 breaths. Raise the head and then tilt the head back, relaxing into the stretch. Repeat this 3 times. While the head is back the mouth can be opened wide and then closed 3 times for an extra stretch through the throat.

SIDE TO SIDE

1 Turn the head to the right and look over the right shoulder. Hold the position for 3 breaths and then turn to the left to repeat the exercise. The shoulders should be relaxed. Repeat this 3 times each side.

HEAD TO THE SHOULDER

1 Lower the head towards the right shoulder and hold this position while you breathe. Then repeat the exercise, taking the head towards the left shoulder. Do not force the head over too far, or allow any strain in the neck or the shoulders. Repeat this 3 times.

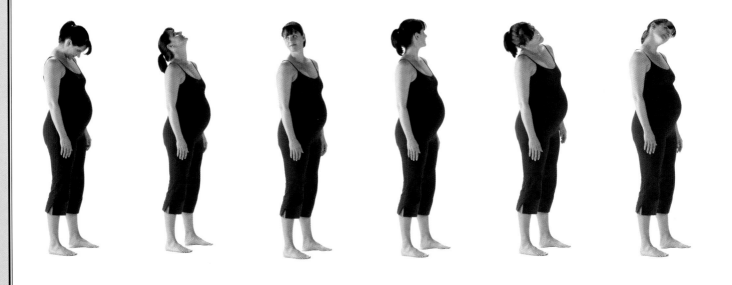

ROLLING THE SHOULDERS

SKANDHACHAKRA

Benefits *Rolling the shoulders works deeply through the muscles of the upper back and will help to release tightness from the upper body giving greater flexibility and suppleness in the shoulders.*

1 Stand with the body relaxed and the feet a little apart, fingertips are on the shoulders. Breathe in and bring the elbows together at the centre of the chest and raise them up above the head.

2 As you breathe out take the elbows back to rotate the shoulders and open up through the chest for a full expansion.

3 This can be repeated 5 times. When the exercise is completed shake the arms lightly.

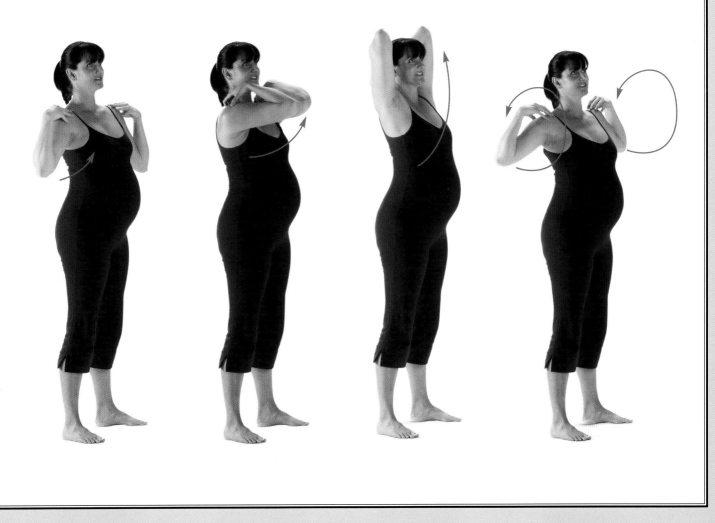

TREE BALANCE

VRIKSASANA

Benefits *The Tree is a lovely posture for giving poise and grace to the body especially during pregnancy when the weight of the body changes so much. This posture also strengthens the supporting leg and greatly improves concentration. Traditionally the leg is held either on the side of the inner thigh, or resting in front of the thigh. However, it is acceptable to simply place the foot on top of the supporting foot, as the purpose of this posture is to improve balance rather than focus on where the foot is positioned.*

1 Stand with the body relaxed and before lifting the foot from the floor choose a stationary object to focus on, as this will help you to concentrate and make it easier to balance.

2 Place the right foot either on top of the left foot, beside the left thigh, or in front of the thigh. The hands are either in the prayer position with the palms joined at the centre of the chest or raised above the head with the arms straight and the palms together. Once the position has been established relax the supporting foot. If the leg is held high on the thigh, gently move the knee back slightly to open up more deeply into the hip. Relax into the pose and feel you are stretching up from the foot right through to the top of the head, so that the body feels tall and balanced.

3 Hold this final position for between 5 and 9 breaths.

4 Lower the leg and shake the legs before repeating the Tree Balance on the left leg. Remember to hold both sides for an equal number of breaths.

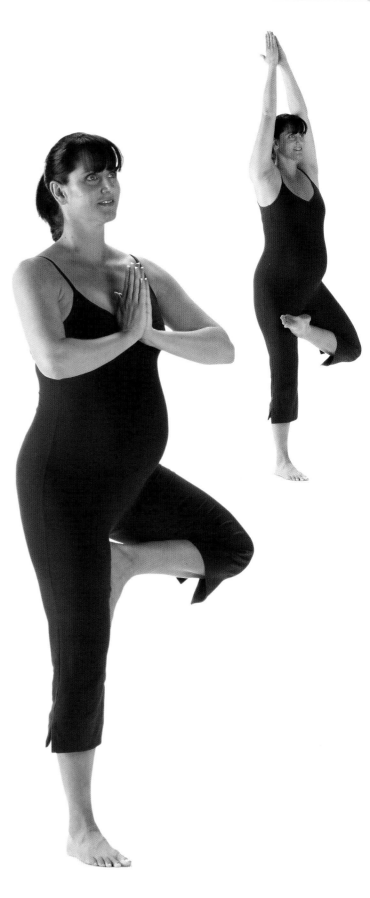

HEAVENLY STRETCH

TADASANA

Benefits *This posture works deeply into the muscles of the feet and the lower legs as you balance on the toes. A strong stretch will also be felt in the sides of the body, whilst concentration and steadiness will be improved. If you find it too difficult to balance on the toes this can be practised on the flat feet instead.*

This can be repeated up to 5 times and can be practised in two ways:
(i) Breathe in as you come up onto the toes, then breathe out as the feet come to the floor and the arms are lowered
(ii) For a deeper stretch and longer balance, inhale as you come into the stretch, hold the balance while breathing 3 or 4 times. Return to a standing position as you exhale.

1 Stand with the feet together and the hands joined in front of the body. Focus on a stationary object before you begin.

2 Raise the hands to the throat then turn the palms upwards for the stretch above the head, and come up onto the toes. Hold the balance while stretching the hands to the ceiling, the shoulders are relaxed.

3 Come back onto the feet as the hands are lowered, turning them again at the throat.

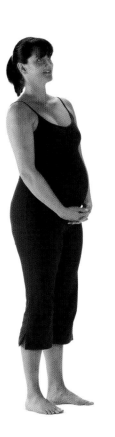
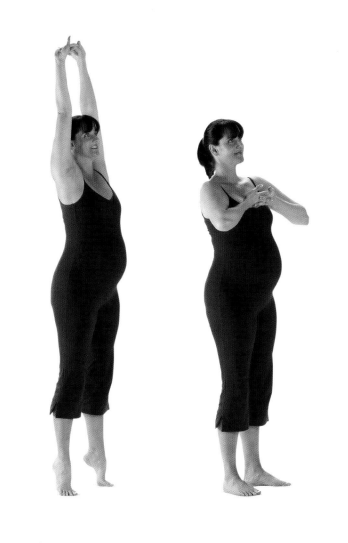

STANDING WIDE LEG STRETCHES

PRASAVITA PADOTTANASANA

Benefits *These postures offer many important benefits for pregnancy either in the full posture or the modified variations. The wide leg stretches work deeply into the inner thigh muscles and pelvis, bringing suppleness and increased flexibility in preparation for childbirth. The lower back is also opened and receives a lovely stretch. They are ideal if you are experiencing lower back or pelvic discomfort, while in the last weeks before delivery the heaviness of your pregnancy can be very uncomfortable and this position takes the weight 'away' from your body for some welcome light relief.*

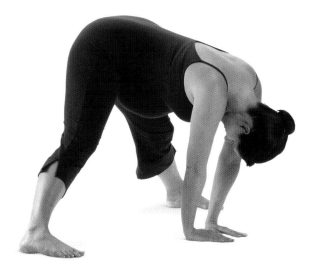

1 The legs are as wide as possible with the feet to the front so that you feel you can relax into the stretch in complete comfort.

2 Place the hands on a low stool and relax into that position, or lower the hands to the knees or the lower legs. At this point the head is still in line with the back and you are looking straight ahead. If you have high or low blood pressure or feel dizzy with the head down, remain in this position so that your head is level with your body.

3 Lower the head down and rest the hands on the ankles or on the floor.

4 Once in your final pose relax and breathe gently, holding this for 5 breaths.

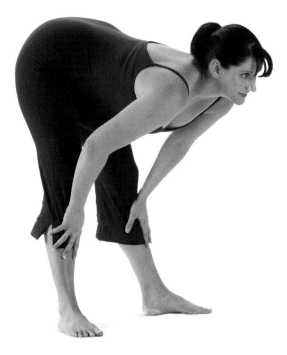

5 When returning to the standing position, come to the halfway point first and stabilise yourself there before returning slowly to a standing position. Bring the legs together and shake them lightly. Always remember it is better to be as relaxed as possible in the posture rather than attempting to stretch too far, where discomfort will be felt rather than the benefits.

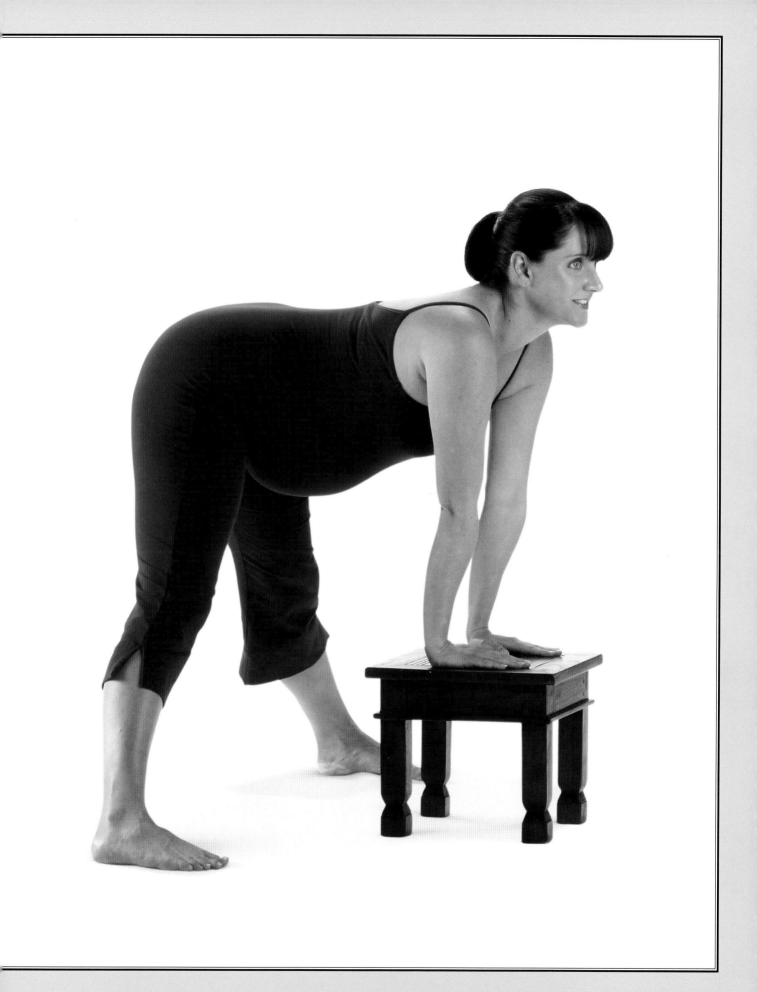

PELVIC ROCKING

Benefits *Pelvic rocking is an effective way to relax deeply into the lower body and free tightness from the hips and pelvic areas. For these reasons it is often suggested during labour to increase relaxation and to enable gravity to assist with the baby's journey through the birth canal.*

1 Stand with the feet about hip-distance apart, or a little wider if you prefer, and slowly move the body in big slow circles, rotating the hips, 5 or more times one way and then the other. This can be continued for as long as desired.

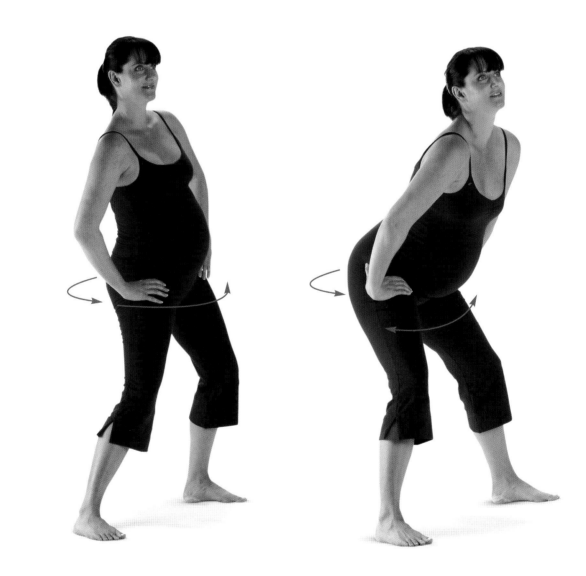

DEEP STANDING SQUAT

UTTHANASANA

Benefits *This is a very strong posture that will strengthen and tone the muscles of the thighs, the lower back and the pelvic areas. Like the Wide Leg Stretches and Squatting it is ideal for pregnancy and in preparation for birth. It is important not to strain or over-exert yourself in this deep squat – your stamina and endurance will determine how long you can remain in the final position. If you have a lower back weakness this is an important exercise to practise regularly as it will improve strength in this area.*

1 Stand with the feet hip-distance apart or wider, with the feet facing to the front.

2 Breathe in to prepare and breathe out to move into the squat. The upper body is relaxed. The hips and pelvis should be tilted forward rather than back, which will increase the depth of the position and the exertion required but ultimately is more valuable and strengthening. Breathe quietly while the position is held.

3 Either remain in the static pose or move slowly from side to side before returning to the standing position. Shake the legs on completing the pose. For a deeper inner-thigh stretch rest the elbows on the knees.

NOTE
Over-exertion in this posture can cause shaky legs, fatigue and soreness. The static position is not recommended if you are feeling tired or weak.

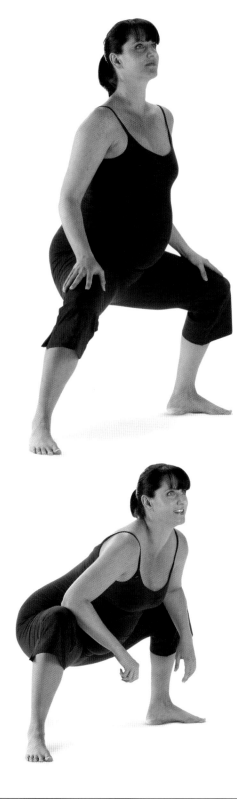

EASY SPINAL TWIST

KATI CHAKRASANA

Benefits *This easy twist is a gentle and effective way to loosen the back and improve flexibility. With regular practice it will free the back from tension and tightness.*

1 Stand with the feet hip-distance apart and raise the arms to the side while breathing in.

2 Twist to the right and wrap the arms around the body as you breathe out. Hold this position while you breathe.

3 Breathe in and return to the front with the arms out to the side. Breathe out and twist to the left. This can be repeated 5 or more times on each side. To finish you can swing a little faster 5 times in each direction.

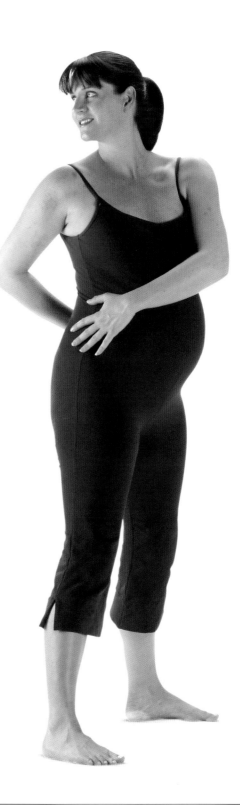

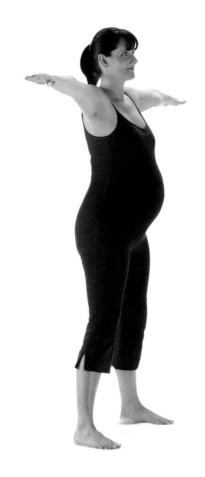

POSE OF TWO ANGLES

DWI KONASANA

Benefits *Tension is often held between the shoulder blades. This posture is a wonderful way to ease that tension and remove stiffness from the shoulders and the neck. The precautions suggested for all the standing, head-down postures are applicable for this posture also (see Precautions, p.6).*

1 Stand with the feet hip-distance apart, the feet facing the front and the hands joined behind the back.

2 Breathe in to prepare and as you breathe out bend as far forward as you can, with the top of the head in line with the floor and the arms raised above your back.

3 Hold this position for 5 breaths before returning slowly to a standing position, as you breathe in.

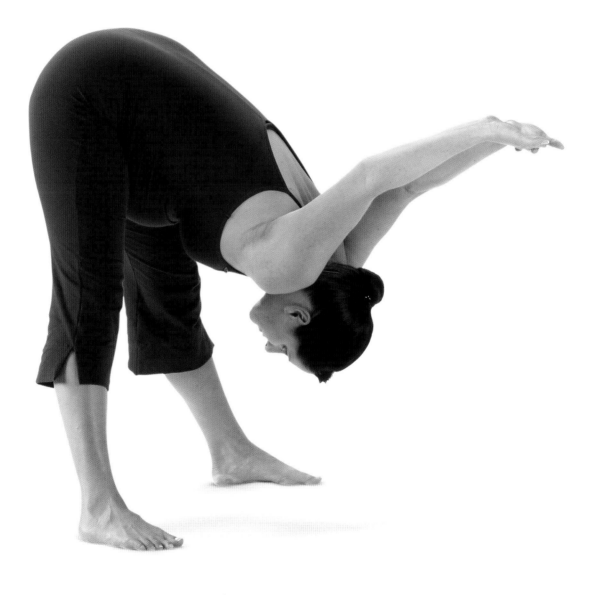

WARRIOR POSE 1 & 2

VIRABHADRASANA

Benefits *The Warrior Poses 1 and 2 both help to build strength and stamina in the whole body while increasing tone to the leg muscles and the arms. The poses are considered quite dynamic in nature as they require a reasonable level of fitness if they are to be held for any length of time, therefore it is important to only remain in the final position while you are relaxed and are not straining.*

WARRIOR 1

1 Stand with the legs wide and the feet to the front.

2 Turn the right foot to the right, keeping the hips and shoulders square to the front.

3 Turn the head to the right and breathe in while raising the arms, stretching through to the fingertips.

4 Breathe out and bend the right knee and hold the pose for 5 breaths or more.
If you find this easy, bend the knee more and move deeper into the pose.

5 Breathe in to return to the standing position and lower the arms as you breathe out.

6 Rest before repeating this to the other side.

WARRIOR 2

1 Stand with the legs wide and the feet to the front and turn the body to the right. The hands are in the prayer position at the centre of the chest.

2 Breathe in to prepare. Breathe out and bend the right leg, feeling the strength in the right thigh muscle and the weight on the outside of the left foot. Hold this for 5 breaths, or longer, before breathing in, straightening the leg and returning to the centre front. Relax before repeating this to the left.

3 Shake the legs and rest on completing the posture.

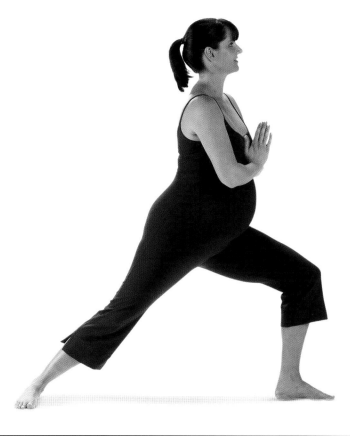

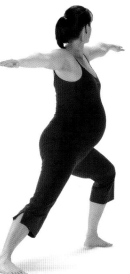

TRIANGLE POSE 1 & 2
Trikonasana

Benefits *A deep stretch is felt through the side of the body and the inner thigh, while a gentle contraction is felt as you lean to each side. The digestive system benefits from the light compression and the waist is lightly firmed and toned. This exercise is also known as the Side Bend Pose.*

TRIANGLE POSE 1

1 Stand with the legs wide and the feet to the front, the arms resting beside the body.

2 Turn the right foot to the right and breathe in as you raise the arms to shoulder height.

3 Breathe out and lean to the right, resting the right hand on the right leg and raise the left arm, look up at the left hand. Relax into the position, holding it for 5 breaths or longer. Some people prefer not to look up finding it easier to look straight ahead. The right knee can be bent instead of being held straight.

4 To return to the standing position breathe in and lower the arms as you breathe out.

5 Repeat this bending to the left.

TRIANGLE POSE 2

1 Repeat Steps 1 and 2 of the previous posture.

2 Breathe out and bend the right knee and rest the right elbow on the knee. Stretch the left arm across the body to feel a full stretch through the left side of the body from the hip to the fingertips. Hold this for 5 breaths before returning to the standing position as you breathe in, lower the arms as you breathe out.

3 Repeat this to the left. On completing the posture, bring the feet together and shake the legs lightly.

POSE OF THE CHILD (MODIFIED FOR PREGNANCY)

SISHUASANA

Benefits *The modified Child Pose is probably the most relaxing and enjoyable of all yoga postures to use during your pregnancy and in childbirth.*

This posture has a relaxing influence on the mind and a very calming effect on the emotions and is especially valuable during times of stress. Physically it relaxes the back and is the position of choice if lower back problems or pelvic discomfort are experienced.

If you are in labour on the hands and knees this is an ideal position to rest in after a contraction and for relaxing massage during this time. It is often used during labour as the ideal pose if you have back pain, especially if

the baby is in the posterior position. If you have swollen feet or varicose veins one or two thick cushions placed in between the legs will enable you to stay in this pose in complete comfort and it can easily be adjusted to suit the needs of all women simply by using cushions or even a bean bag.

1 Sit on the feet with the toes together and the knees comfortably apart, using cushions where needed for complete comfort. There are three positions to choose from:
  (i) the head resting on the hands (ii) the chin rests in the hands (iii) the arms stretched forward with the forehead on the floor. Because of this posture's many benefits it is worthwhile finding the most comfortable position for complete relaxation.

Rest and relax deeply into the pose following the natural breath. This pose can be held for as long as desired.

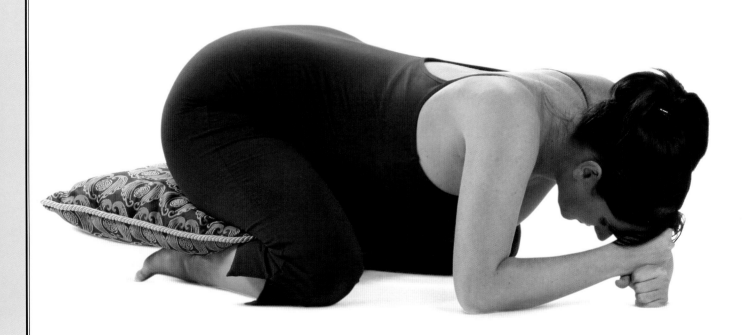

CAT POSE

MARJARIASANA

Benefits *The Cat is an excellent posture for all pregnant women as is relaxes the pelvis and relieves lower back discomfort. It works directly on the female reproductive system and is an ideal exercise to practise throughout the entire pregnancy.*

1 Come onto the hands and the knees, the knees hip-distance apart and the hands shoulder- distance apart. The position is balanced and relaxed.

2 Position 1. Breathe in and look ahead remembering to keep the back straight.

3 Position 2. Breathe out while arching the back to tilt the pelvis forward. The arms remain straight throughout.

4 Repeat this movement 5 or more times remembering to tighten the pelvic floor muscles as you breathe out.

5 On completion shake the hands and rest in the modified Pose of the Child or do Pelvic Rocking (see p. 57).

NOTE

During pregnancy the back is held straight in Position 1, rather than arched as is recommended when not pregnant.

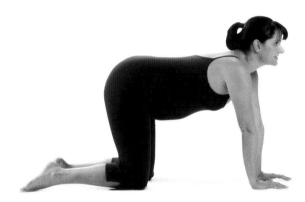

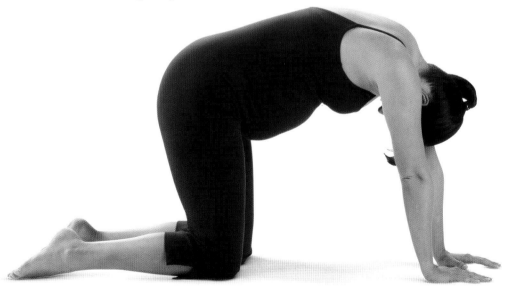

TIGER POSE

VYAGHRASANA

Benefits *Lower back pain can be a major problem during pregnancy and the Tiger is another excellent posture that helps alleviate the problem and in some cases will prevent it becoming worse as the pregnancy progresses. This exercise is especially useful if you suffer from sciatica, as it gently stretches the leg and hip thereby reducing the discomfort considerably. It is similar to the Cat, having a massaging effect on the pelvis, and is therefore highly recommended for pregnant women to practise as regularly as possible.*

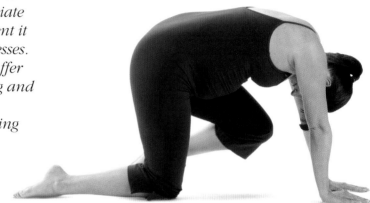

1 Rest on the hands and the knees with the back straight.

2 Breathe in and raise the right leg, the knee can be slightly bent. Look up as the leg is raised.

3 Breathe out and bring the knee in towards the face.

4 Repeat this exercise 5 times with the right leg and 5 times with the left leg. Rest in between each side and shake the hands lightly. Relax into the Pose of the Child (see p. 26) or Pelvic Rocking (see p. 57), on completion.

Note: *I have found that between 30 and 35 weeks some women find the Tiger can become uncomfortable to do, in which case, it is best to discontinue for a few weeks before commencing it again later on.*

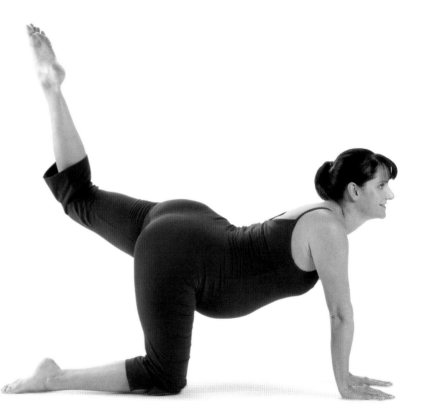

Floor Exercises
Exercises for the Feet

Benefits *These gentle exercises improve circulation to the feet and the ankles and increase flexibility. During pregnancy it is not uncommon for the feet and ankles to swell, especially during the summer months, and these exercises are an effective way of gaining some relief from the discomfort.*

1 Sit on a cushion with the legs straight in front of you and place the hands behind the back for support.

2 Flex the feet up and then point the toes down, holding each position for about 5 seconds. Repeat the exercise 3 times.

3 Rotate the feet in big, slow circles 5 times to the right and then 5 times to the left. For the best results make these movements quite strong and firm where the stretch is felt into the lower legs.

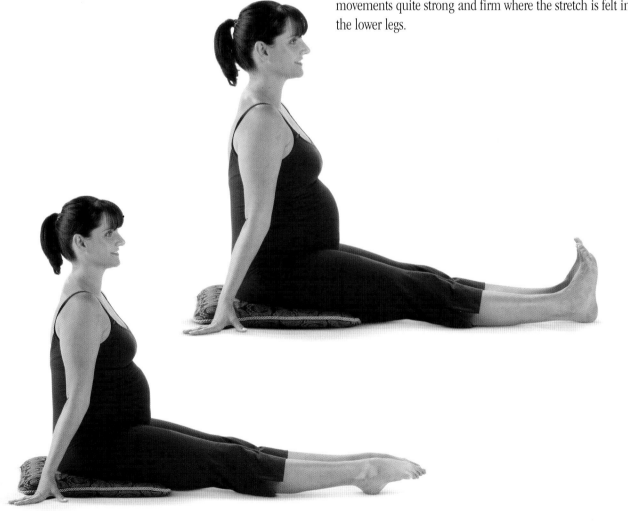

HIP ROTATION

SHONI CHAKRA

Benefits *Tightness and stiffness are reduced as the hip joint is gently rotated. The Hip Rotation improves flexibility and is an ideal preparation pose for the Butterfly, the Squatting postures and the Seated Wide Leg Stretches.*

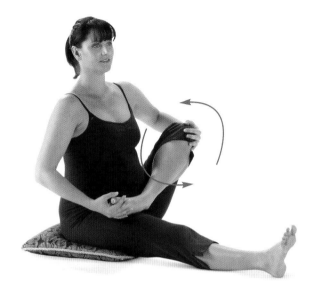

1 Sit on the floor with a cushion for extra support. Bend the right leg and hold onto the right knee and foot, and make big slow circles with the leg, repeating this 5 times one way and 5 times the other way. At first this might feel a bit awkward but in time it will become easier. As a guideline think about drawing big circles with the knee rather than focusing on the hip. Repeat this with the left leg.

HALF BUTTERFLY

Benefits *This posture has similar benefits to the Hip Rotation and loosens the hip in preparation for the Full Butterfly Pose.*

1 Sit comfortably on a cushion and bend the right leg, placing the right foot either on top of the thigh or beside the right inner thigh.

2 Lightly bounce the knee up and down 9 times before releasing the foot. Shake the leg lightly and then repeat this same movement with the left leg.

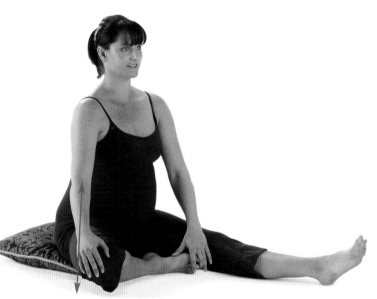

FULL BUTTERFLY

BADDHAKONASANA

Benefits *The Butterfly is considered one of the most important exercises for pregnant women as it prepares the areas of the body that are most involved in childbirth, increasing suppleness, strength and improving flexibility. The muscles of the inner thighs are toned and the whole pelvic region is opened in preparation for childbirth. If you are not very flexible in this position take care not to over-extend or force the knees down. You will find with continued practice your flexibility increases quite quickly.*

1 Sit on a cushion with the back straight and bring the soles of the feet together. Hold onto the feet and gently bounce the knees up and down, like the wings of a butterfly. This can be repeated for as long as you desire.

2 Place the hands behind the back and lean back slightly. The knees will move down naturally for a lovely open stretch. Hold the legs still in this position as you relax and breathe into the stretch.

3 When you have completed the pose stretch the legs to the front and shake them lightly.

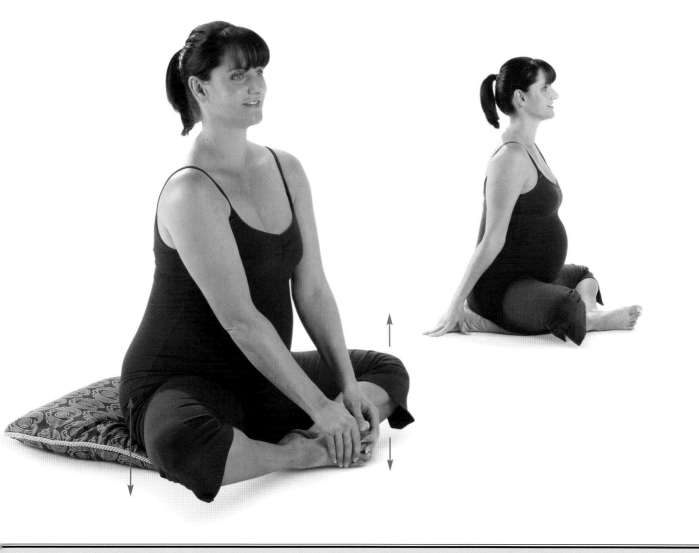

BUTTERFLY POSE

Benefits *This is considered to be one of the most important exercises for pregnant women as the emphasis is on working deeply into the whole pelvic area. The benefits are similar to the previous exercise but to a much greater degree – flexibility, suppleness and tone are increased in the pelvis while the back is lightly stretched. Deeper breathing is also encouraged as you inhale and stretch up through the back. The lower back receives a lovely open stretch as you breathe out to bend forward.*

1 Sit on a cushion with the soles of the feet together and the hands on the feet.

2 Breathe in, stretch through the back and look up, at the same time gently pushing the knees down as far as is comfortable.

3 Breathe out and lean forward. Relax the shoulders and bring the head towards the feet, as the arms gently push the knees down. The purpose of this pose is to receive all the potential benefits, not how far forward you are able to bend, as your size, how you are carrying the baby and your general flexibility will determine how far you are able to move forward in comfort.

4 Repeat this sequence 5 times.

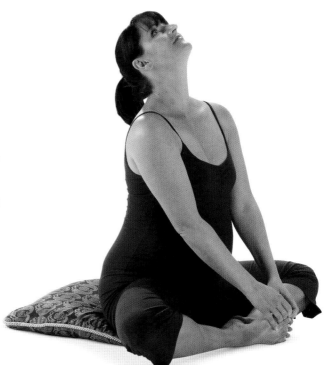

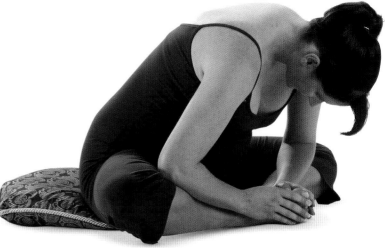

SLEEPING TORTOISE (MODIFIED FOR PREGNANCY)

SUPTA KURMASANA

Benefits *The Sleeping Tortoise is a valuable relaxation pose that can be practised throughout the pregnancy, either in its full position, or to a lesser degree as your pregnancy progresses. How comfortable you are really depends on the individual and if you do not enjoy it now, it is one to remember after the birth for rest and relaxation. This posture has a very calming influence on an unsettled mind and is excellent in times of stress and tension. Physically it releases tension and tightness from the neck and the shoulders, and relaxes deeply through the lower back and is an excellent pose if you are suffering from upper-body discomfort.*

1 Sit on a cushion with the soles of the feet together in the Butterfly Pose (see opposite) and then move the feet a little further away from the body.

2 Rest as far forward as you can, making sure that the head, neck and shoulders are completely relaxed. The hands are either on top of the feet or tucked under the legs.

3 Close your eyes and relax into this pose following the natural breath. Your head will gradually come closer to the feet the longer you remain in the pose and the more relaxed, physically and emotionally, you will become. Even if you are only able to move a little way forward you will still notice these benefits.

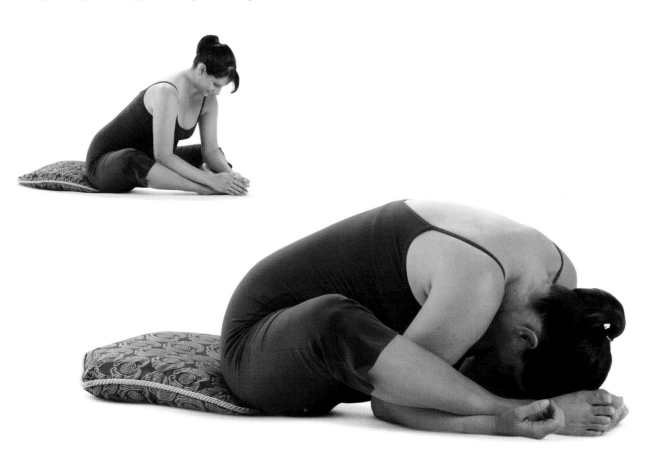

SEATED WIDE LEG STRETCH

PAVISTHA KONASANA

Benefits *The Seated Wide Leg Stretch works deeply into the inner thigh muscles and is excellent to practise during pregnancy in preparation for birth. However it is important to be aware that this is not an easy pose. You might find these muscles are tight and you have little flexibility, so in the next three postures only stretch as far as you can in complete comfort and without straining. Sitting on one or two cushions is helpful, as the pelvis is tilted forward making it easier to sit up straight, and also giving you more room under the ribs, especially if you are carrying the baby high. If you have a lower back injury the forward-bending postures are not recommended.*

NOTE

After bending forward it is always important to practise a suitable counter-pose to relieve the back, either Pelvic Rocking (see p. 57), massaging the back (see p. 56), or resting in the Pose of the Child (see p. 26).

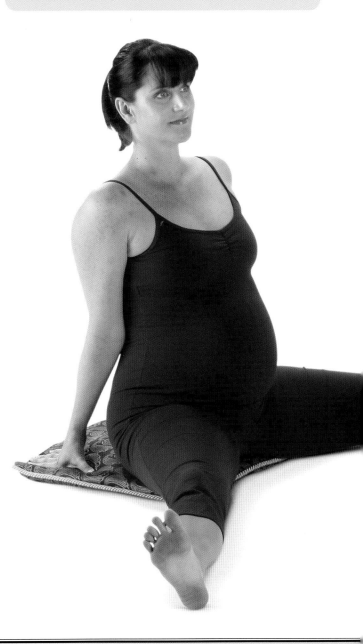

1 Make yourself comfortable sitting on cushions with the legs as wide as possible.

2 Lean forward and relax into this position with the head down and the shoulders relaxed. How far forward you move is not important – if it is too uncomfortable just relax into the seated position. Breathe quietly and rest there for 5 or more breaths.

3 Breathe in to prepare, then extend over the right leg as you breathe out, coming as far over the leg as you can, relaxing in complete comfort for 5 breaths. The arms are relaxed and are slightly bent to prevent tension in the shoulders.

4 Breathe in to return to the seated position and then repeat the stretch over the left leg. One side might be easier than the other due to the position of the baby and suppleness in your spine.

5 On completing the pose bring the legs together and shake them lightly.

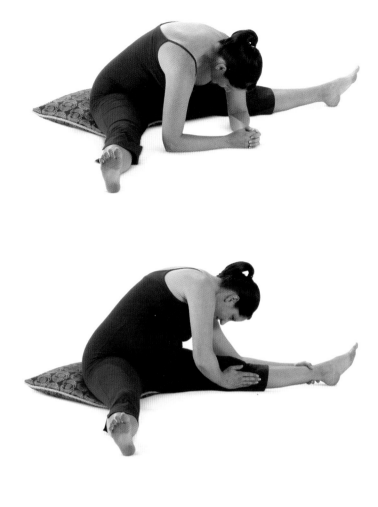

HEAD TO KNEE POSE

JANU SIRSHASANA

1 Sit on a cushion with the right leg straight and the left leg bent.

2 Breathe in to prepare then breathe out as you bring the body towards the leg, the head is relaxed towards the leg. Hold this for 5 breaths before returning to a seated position. It is important to be very relaxed in the final position, with only a light stretch felt in the hamstring muscles and the lower back.

3 Change legs and repeat this to the other side.

4 On completing the pose, rest in a counter-pose as recommended for the Seated Wide Leg Stretch (see note opposite).

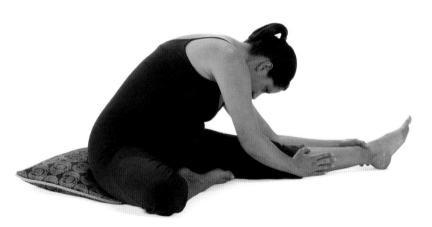

SPINAL TWISTS

MATSYENDRASANA

The Spinal Twists are an important group of postures that should be included in all your yoga sessions because of the significant benefits they provide for the whole body, physically and emotionally. The spinal column runs the length of the body, from the atlas at the top of the spine to the tail bone and is part of the body's complex nervous system. This can be divided into two interdependent parts: the central nervous system, which includes the brain and the spinal cord, and the peripheral nervous system, which directs messages from the brain, via the spinal column throughout the body. Together they enable you to function in day-to-day life – to think, to breathe, to move, either consciously or unconsciously.

This incredible system of tiny nerves reaches every part of the body and our physical and emotional health are dependent on them functioning efficiently and calmly. In yoga the Spinal Twists are essential as they have a valuable influence on the physical body, especially the back and the spinal column while they also encourage mental and emotional stability and wellbeing.

From a physical perspective, when these poses are done regularly the back becomes relaxed and freed from tightness, tension and rigidity so that suppleness and flexibility are greatly improved. Frequent practice can help to alleviate soreness and mild injury in the muscles and when practised correctly the alignment of the whole spinal column can be improved. When these Yoga postures are used in conjunction with other therapies healing often occurs much faster and with lasting results. Because they work deeply through the middle of the body they also have a positive influence on maintaining optimum health in the digestive system and therefore improve digestive function.

The Spinal Twists have a calming effect on the mind and the emotions. When they are practised with a relaxed mind, with awareness of the natural breath and in a comfortable posture they become meditative and peaceful, positively affecting the whole person. Performed in this way, even the most gentle twist will instantly improve your sense of balance and composure.

Follow these guidelines for all the seated twists.

1 Always sit with the back straight and completely relaxed, before commencing and while holding the posture.

2 Breathe in to prepare, then turn into the twist as you breathe out, holding the twist for an equal number of breaths on each side. Breathe in to come out of the twist.

3 For extra comfort, sitting on a cushion will help to keep the back straight and will elevate the pelvis, so you are twisting correctly from the tail bone right through to the top of the neck. The benefits will be felt through the length of the spinal column.

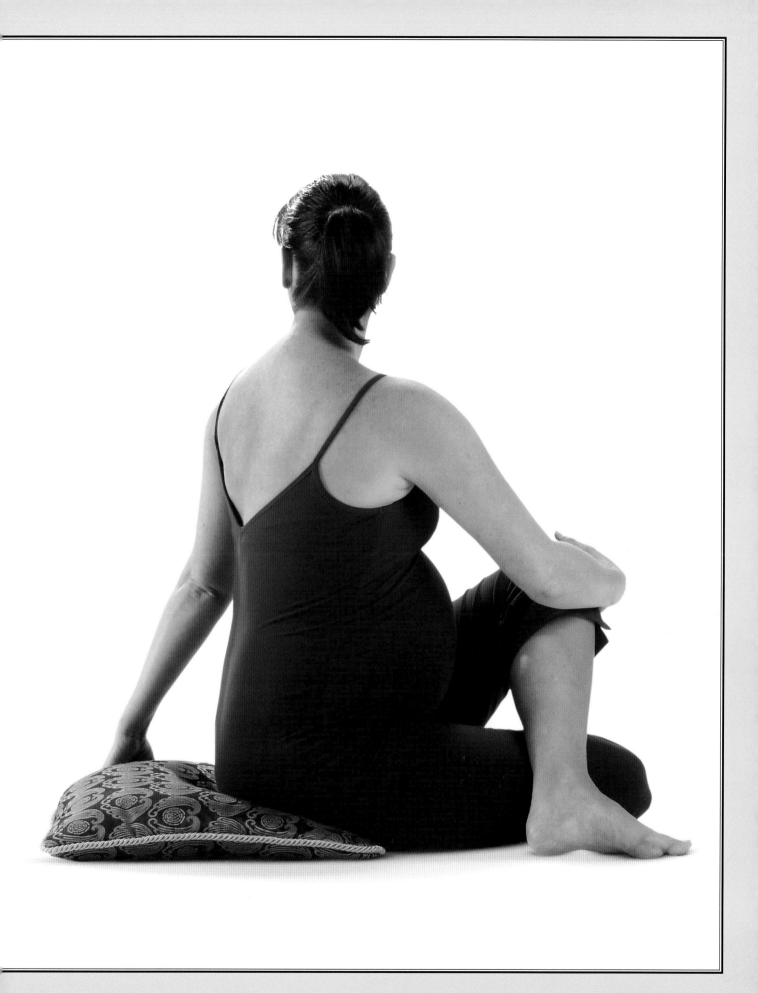

EASY SPINAL TWIST 1

MERU WAKRASANA

1 Sit on a cushion with the legs to the front, the back straight and relaxed.

2 Place the right hand under the left knee, the left hand rests behind the back to support the back and keep the spine straight.

3 Breathe in to prepare, then as you breathe out turn the head and shoulders to the left, holding the pose for 5 breaths or longer if desired.

4 Breathe in to return to the centre front and repeat the twist to the right.

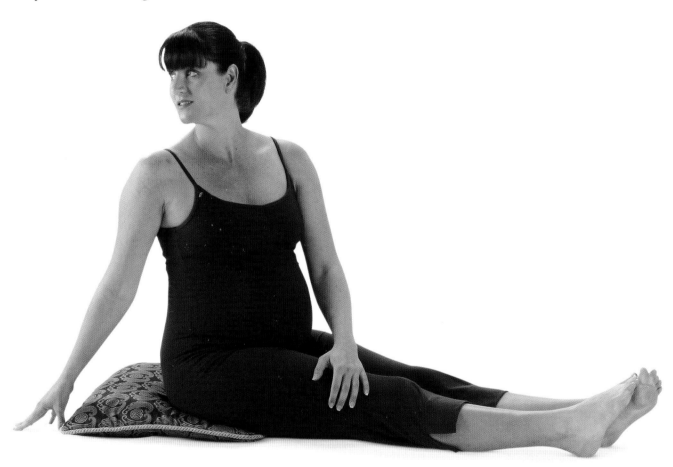

EASY SPINAL TWIST 2

1 Begin as you did for the previous posture.

2 Bend the right leg and place the right foot on the outside of the left leg.

3 The right arm rests on the inside of the right lower leg and the hand is on the foot. The left hand is behind the back for support.

4 Breathe in and as you breathe out turn and look over the left shoulder, gently pushing the arm against the right leg to assist the twist to the left. Relax into the pose for 5 or more breaths.

5 Return to the centre front and repeat this to the other side by reversing all the instructions.

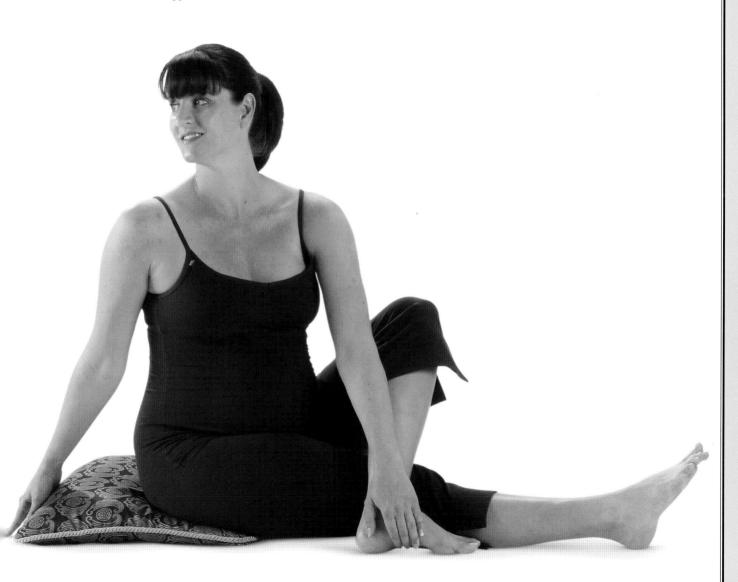

CROSSED LEG SPINAL TWISTS 1 & 2

CROSSED LEG TWIST

1 Sit on a cushion with both legs crossed, the spine straight and the back relaxed.

2 As you turn to the left place the right hand on the left knee and the left hand behind the back. Hold this position for 5 breaths or more before returning to the centre front.

3 Repeat the twist turning to the right and reversing all the instructions.

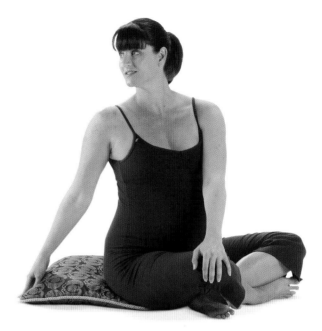

HALF-CROSSED LEG TWIST

1 Prepare as you did for the previous posture.

2 Bend the right leg back so that the foot rests beside the right hip.

3 Place the right hand on the left knee and the left hand behind the back or on the floor. Keep the back relaxed and straight.

4 Look over the left shoulder and relax into the twist for 5 breaths or more.

5 Return to the centre front and reverse the instructions so that the left leg is folded back and you turn to the right. This spinal twist is often preferred to all other seated spinal twists, as it gives a lovely open stretch through the abdomen and a deeper expansion through the hip.

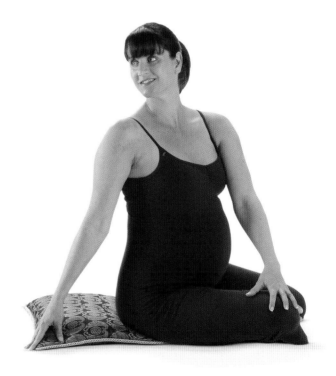

HALF SPINAL TWIST
(MODIFIED FOR PREGNANCY)

1 Sit on a cushion with the spine straight and the legs crossed.

2 Place the right foot in front of the left knee, so you are sitting balanced on the legs and the buttocks.

3 The right hand is resting on the inside of the right lower leg and the left hand is on the floor behind the back.

4 Breathe in to prepare, then as you breathe out turn to the left and relax into this lovely posture. If you find you are tipping over towards the left hip, place an extra cushion under the hip so that you are sitting balanced and steady. Hold the final position for 5 breaths or more before returning to the front, shaking the legs lightly if you need to.

5 Repeat the twist with the left leg in front and the body turning to the right.

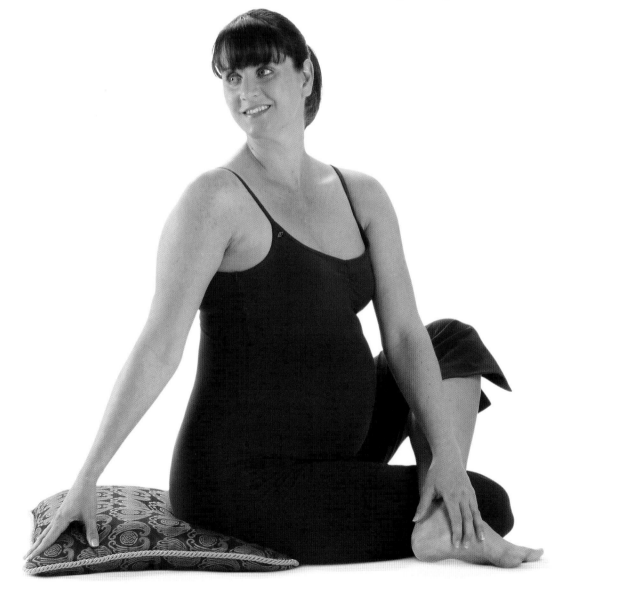

FULL SPINAL TWIST (MODIFIED FOR PREGNANCY)

ARDHA MATSYENDRASANA

Benefits   *The Full Spinal Twist has been modified slightly for pregnancy to provide all its benefits, but with the most comfort. As your pregnancy progresses and your size and shape change you will probably not want to twist as far and the position of the hand might alter slightly too. For these reasons you will need to adapt the posture to suit your individual needs. If the full twist becomes too uncomfortable then it would be preferable to practise one of the easier ones instead.*

1 Proceed as you did for the previous posture, adjusting your cushions for comfort and stability.

2 The right leg is over the left and for the full pose you will turn to the right, placing the left hand either on the right knee or the left knee. The right hand is behind the back. Look over the right shoulder and relax into the twist while you take 5 or more breaths. The left arm and shoulder should not be tight or tense.

3 When you have completed the twist return to the front. Change the legs so that the left leg is front of the right and you turn to the left. Stay in the posture for the same number of breaths on each side.

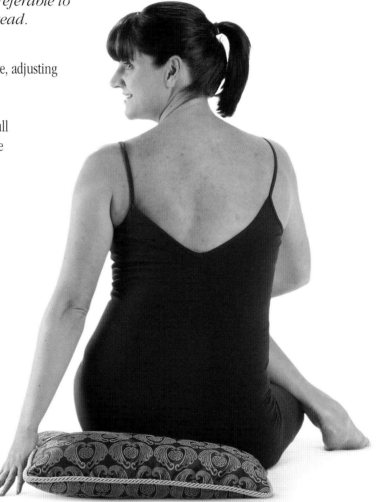

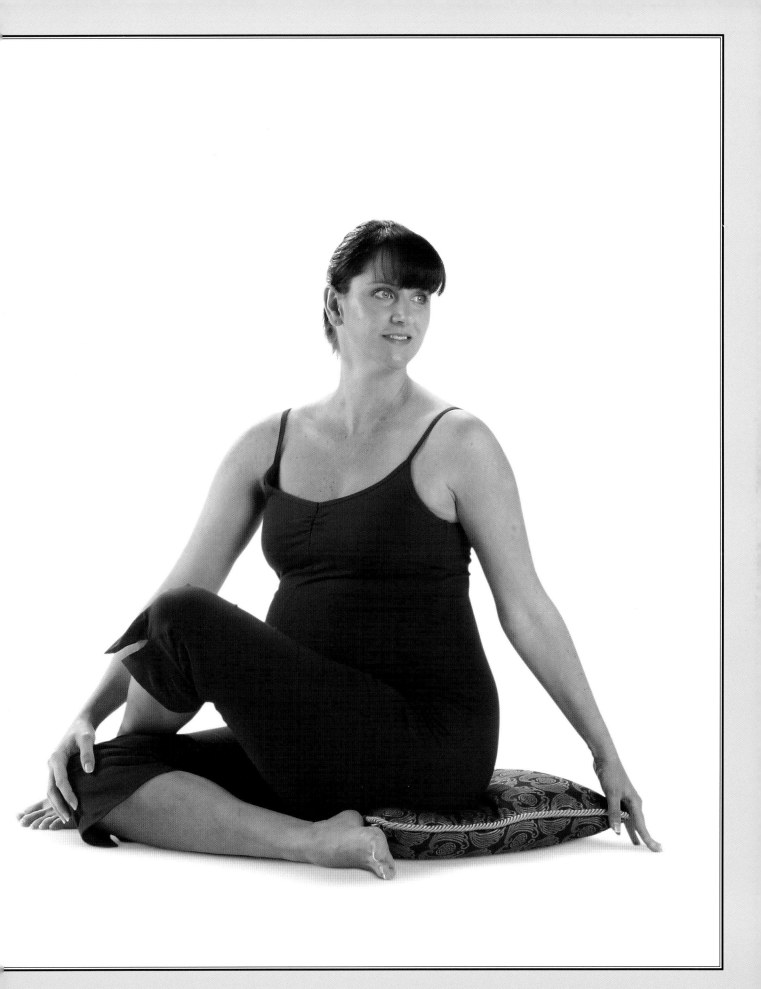

Arm Exercises
Head of the Cow
Gomukhasana

Benefits *Tension and tightness are often held in the upper body, especially the shoulders and the upper back, however the upper arms can also be very tight. This posture works deeply into all these muscles, improving suppleness and mobility. It is usually easier to do this exercise on one side of the body than the other, but with continued practice an equal level of flexibility will soon be felt. One of the aims of yoga is to establish balance and equilibrium in all parts of the body.*

1 Sit with the back straight, either with the legs crossed or in a chair for more comfort.

2 Raise the left arm as high up the centre of the back as possible, being aware that the shoulder is relaxed.

3 Bend the right arm over the right shoulder and reach down to hold onto the left hand, making sure the elbow is back for a full stretch in the upper arm. If you are not able to reach your hand, a length of rope can be used to fill the gap. Once you are in the final position relax the upper body and the arms, and hold the pose for 5 breaths.

4 Lower the arms and shake them lightly before repeating this exercise to the other side, reversing all the instructions.

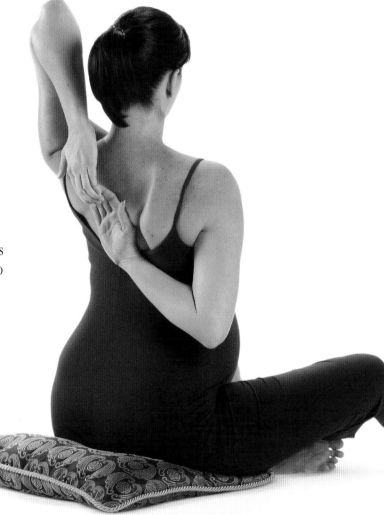

FROG POSE & ARM EXERCISES
Mandukasana

Benefits *These are two separate postures practised together. The Frog Pose gives a lovely inner-thigh stretch and you will find it easy to hold the back straight and relaxed in this position. For extra comfort you can sit on one or two cushions which is required if you have swollen feet, or find the pose too difficult. This pose is not recommended if you have varicose veins and a stool or a low step should be used instead. With the Arm Exercises the arms and shoulders are toned and firmed and the pectoral muscles in the chest also benefit.*

1 Sit on cushions with the toes together and the heels apart, the knees are as wide apart as possible. The spine is straight and the upper body relaxed.

2 Join the palms of the hands above the head in the prayer position. Bend the arms so that the hands rest on top of the head, with the shoulders relaxed.

3 Breathe in and push the hands together while straightening the arms. Breathe out as you lower the hands to the head, again pushing the hands together. Repeat this 5 times. When this is done correctly you will feel it working quite strongly into the muscles of the upper arms, the shoulders and the chest.

4 On completing the pose, lower the arms and shake them lightly.

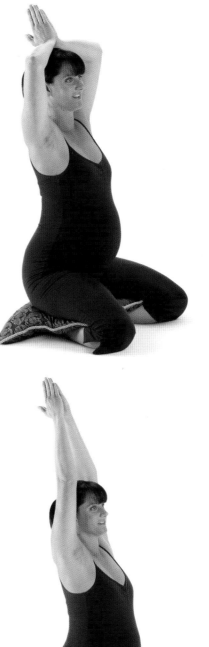

SQUATTING POSES

Women have been using the squatting position or similar for childbirth since ancient times as it works with gravity and makes childbirth so much easier. It is only since Victorian times that the prone position has become more common, adding greatly to women's discomfort.

Fortunately today women have choices and are more aware of the benefits to be gained from being in an upright position to deliver, either in a full squatting position or a supported semi-squat. These positions provide optimum relaxation for the pelvic floor muscles and maximum pressure inside the pelvis. Women who use this position often have an easier time during labour and generally a faster delivery because the contractions are not so intense and the body is at the perfect angle for delivery. Even if the squatting position is not used during labour, regular practice of it during pregnancy is recommended due to the many wonderful benefits it has to offer.

When the squatting exercises and postures are practised regularly they tone and strengthen the pelvic floor muscles and uterus, and circulation is improved to the feet, the legs and the lower body. They encourage the hips and the knees to become more flexible and because squatting reduces the curve in the lower spine they are excellent for relieving lower-back discomfort and pelvic pain, especially sciatica which can be a common problem during pregnancy. As well as this, these exercises massage deeply into the small and large intestine and pelvic area, so they are an excellent way to help overcome constipation, which can be distressing during pregnancy.

Some women find squatting easy to do and can move through all the postures from the full position unsupported where the toes or the flat feet are on the floor. However, if you are very stiff in the legs or the hips, have a knee injury or varicose veins it is recommended that the modifications suggested be followed rather than giving up completely due to discomfort. The benefits are there for you whether you are sitting on a low stool or in the full posture.

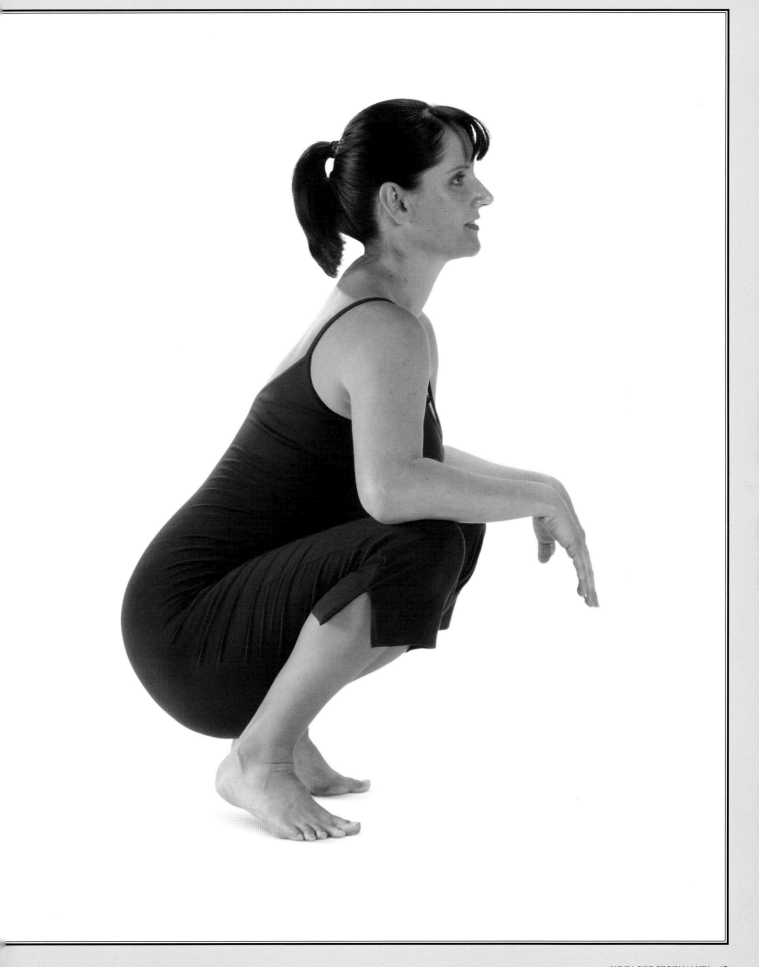

SQUATTING ON A STOOL

This is the best way to practise all the squatting postures if you find the full squat too difficult, due to lack of flexibility or if you have knee problems or varicose veins. You will still receive all the benefits of squatting but without the pressure on the legs, and with much more comfort. Lean forward and gently open the knees wider with the arms, to feel a deeper inner-thigh stretch, remaining there for as long as you wish.

Squatting on a low stool is sometimes used during labour and childbirth because it is comfortable and is an ideal posture for labour as gravity helps the baby move more easily down through the birth canal.

FULL SQUATTING POSE

Depending on your flexibility, the Full Squatting Pose can be done either with the feet flat on the floor or on the toes – both give the same benefits.

1 Come into the full squatting position, either from a standing position or from the floor, with the feet about hip-distance apart. The hands can rest on the floor or if you find squatting easy rest the elbows on the knees.

NOTE

This posture is also very relaxing to do with the lower back resting against the wall, where you lean back and simply relax into the squat. For a deeper stretch into the thighs and the hips join the hands in the prayer position at the centre of the chest and have the elbows on the inside of the knees. Gently press the knees a little wider, making sure that you are relaxed and not straining.

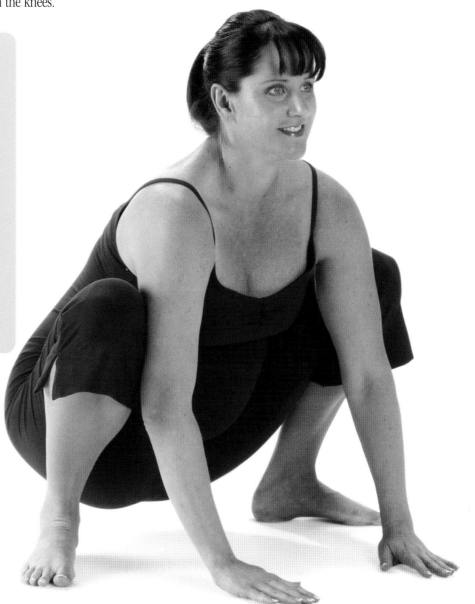

ROCKING FROM SIDE TO SIDE

From the Full Squatting position (see p. 49) move the feet further apart, place the hands on the floor and simply rock slowly from side to side. This is a wonderful exercise to free tightness and stiffness from the feet and the legs and is very relaxing for the lower back. It can also be practised on a stool or a low step for extra comfort.

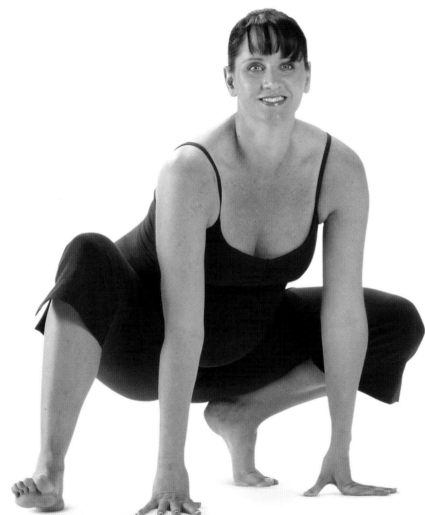

SQUAT & RISE POSE

VAYU NISHKASANA

Benefits *This exercise provides all the benefits of squatting while also giving a deep stretch through the hamstrings. It is excellent for improving circulation to the lower body and the legs. If you don't like the static squatting positions this is a good alternative, as you are continuously moving from a squat to the standing position.*

1 Begin in a squatting position either on the flat feet or on the toes. Rest the hands on the feet.

2 Breathe in and come up to a standing position with the legs straight, the hands rest either on the feet or higher up the legs.

3 Breathe out and relax the head down. If you don't want to have the head down, look ahead instead.

4 Breathe in and look up, breathe out as you come back into the squat. Continue with the exercise keeping the movements in time with the breathing, repeating it 5 times.

5 Rest on completing the exercise and shake the legs.

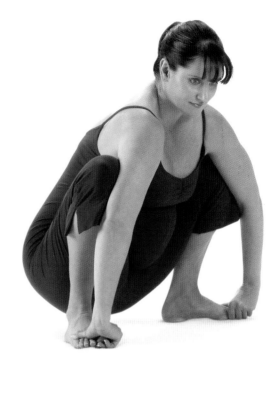

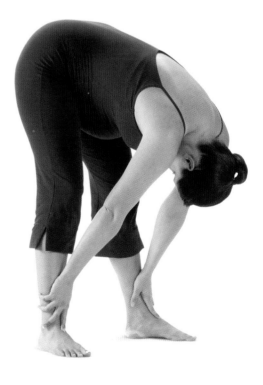

SLOW CHOPPING WOOD

Benefits *Chopping Wood is a dynamic and powerful posture that is valuable for pregnancy as it strengthens the legs, the pelvic area and the lower back. However, it is strenuous and care needs to be taken not to over-exert yourself, especially if you are not very strong in the legs or are feeling fatigued.*

1 Stand with the feet about hip-distance apart, the hands joined in front of the body.

2 Breathe in and raise the arms above the head, stretching through the body.

3 Breathe out as you come into a deep squat, either onto the toes or the flat feet, and lower the arms. Remember to keep the back straight at all times and use the thigh muscles to move up and down. As an alternative to breathing through the nose, breathe out through the mouth.
Repeat this up to 5 times and rest on completion.

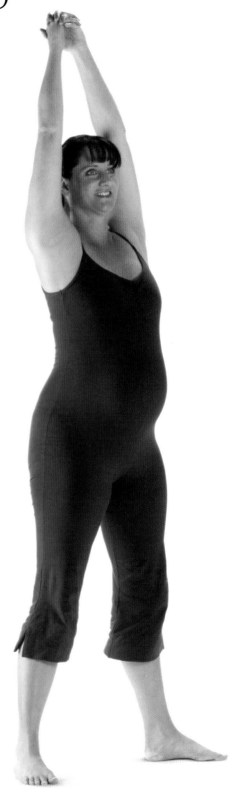

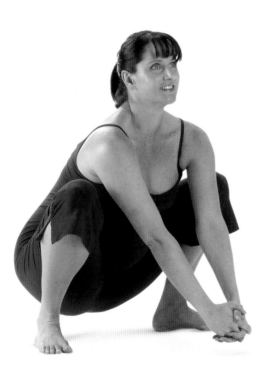

SALUTE POSE

NAMASKARASANA

Benefits *This is a very beneficial posture that provides all the advantages of squatting as well as a deep expansion through the inner thighs, the pelvis and the hips. For these reasons it is highly recommended to practise regularly throughout pregnancy.*

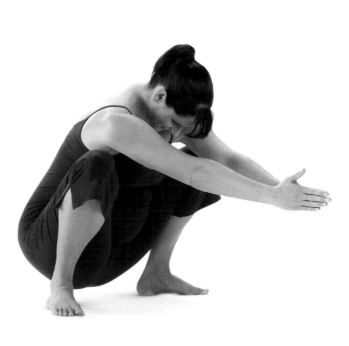

1 Position 1. Come into a comfortable squatting position of your choice. The arms are straight, the palms of the hands joined in the prayer position and the head relaxed down between the shoulders. The outside of the upper arms are on the inside of the knees.

2 Position 2. Breathe in as the hands are brought into the centre of the chest and the elbows gently push the knees wider. Look upwards as this is done and extend through the back.

3 Breathe out and come back to Position 1.

4 Repeat this 5 times and feel a lovely extension through the back, the hips and the whole pelvic area. For extra comfort this posture can be done sitting on a stool, a low step or with the back against the wall.

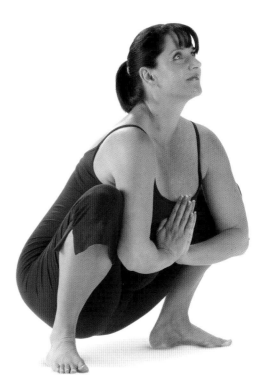

NOTE
When you have completed the squatting exercises, practise Pelvic Rocking on the Hands and Knees (see p. 57) before resting into the Pose of the Child (see p. 26).

LYING ON THE BACK

EASY SPINAL TWIST

SUPTA UDARAKARSHANASANA

Benefits *Both the Easy Spinal Twist and the Full Spinal Twist help to free the back and neck from tension and tightness and greatly improve movement and flexibility. They are an easy way to relieve lower-back discomfort or other problems associated with this area, especially sciatica and hip pain. Because they are practised lying on the back, they are often easier to relax into than the seated postures and are wonderful to do at the end of the day to relieve tension.*

1 Rest on the back with the knees bent and the feet hip-distance apart. Have a cushion under the head and another under the right hip if this is required. Stretch the arms to the sides at shoulder height with the palms facing down on the floor.

2 Breathe in to prepare and as you breathe out take the knees to the right and the head to the left.

3 Breathe in to return to the centre, breathe out and take the knees to the left and the head to the right. Continue with these movements 5 times each side.

4 For a deeper stretch hold the twist for 4 or 5 breaths, repeating this 3 times each side.

NOTE

Before commencing these exercises please refer to the *Precautions* (see p. 6) for the advice recommended for being on your back. Whenever you are either moving onto your back or coming into a sitting position, always move from the side of the body with the knees bent, using the hands for support. This will prevent straining the back and is relevant for these exercises as well as when getting in and out of bed.

FULL SPINAL TWIST

SHAVA UDARAKARSHANASANA

1 Rest on the back with a cushion under the head. Hold the right leg straight and the left leg bent.

2 Place the left foot on the outside of the right knee, the right hand resting on the left knee and the left arm on the floor at shoulder height.

3 Roll over onto the right hip as far as you can and look at the left hand making sure that the shoulder, the hip and the abdomen are not tense in the final position and that the left shoulder remains on the floor. How far the knee comes to the floor will depend on your flexibility – generally one side is more supple than the other.

Once you are completely comfortable close your eyes and relax deeply into the pose for 9 or more breaths.

4 Return to the back and straighten the spine before repeating the twist to the other side, reversing all the instructions.

PELVIC TILT POSE (MODIFIED FOR PREGNANCY)

KANDHARASANA

Benefits *The Pelvic Tilt helps to relieve tension and discomfort from the lower back and is also recommended if you are carrying your baby low and are experiencing pain deep into the pelvis, especially in the last weeks of pregnancy. If you wish to remain in this position for longer, two or three cushions can be placed under the hips which allows you to stay there without any effort for the maximum results.*

NOTE

This exercise is often recommended if the baby is in a transverse or breech position and you are wanting it to move into the head-down position ready for delivery. Although this procedure is often successful it is important to realise that a positive result cannot be guaranteed.

1 Rest on your back with the knees bent, the feet hip-distance apart and as close to the body as possible.

2 Raise the hips as high as you can and place the hands under the hips for extra support. If you feel uncomfortable or slightly breathless lower the hips until you find the most comfortable position.

3 Rest in the final pose for 5 or more breaths.

MASSAGING THE BACK, ROCKING FROM SIDE TO SIDE

Benefits *This is a lovely way to massage the back after practising these exercises. Simply bend the knees and hold the legs close to the body with the hands and gently rock from side to side. This is usually enjoyed by everyone, however, if you are experiencing severe back pain and these movements aggravate the problem it not recommended and Pelvic Rocking (opposite) can be done in its place.*

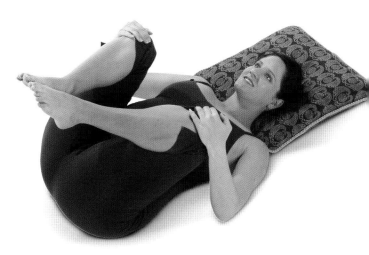

FLAPPING FISH RELAXATION POSE

MATSYA KRIDASANA

Benefits *This is the most comfortable way to rest during pregnancy and is the position of choice for relaxation and while sleeping. It relaxes deeply into the back and stretches through the hip and lower back, helping to relieve sciatic pain and lower-back discomfort.*

In traditional yoga deep relaxation is known as Yoga Nidra and this practice is a wonderfull way to care for yourself during your pregnancy as it is always nourishing and healing. Spending time in a deep relaxation relieves fatigue and reduces the harmful affects of stress thereby improving your energy levels and restoring general well being. During relaxation the mind and the emotions are more detached from he constant flow of unwanted thoughts resulting in increased alertness and clarity and emotional balance.

You will enjoy the benefits from deep relaxation after only 15 or 20 minutes, which can be as refreshing as 2 or 3 hours of deep sleep.

1 Relax on your left side with a cushion under the head, the left arm can be placed under the head and the right hand can rest either on the floor or on the abdomen. The right leg is bent with the knee on the floor, while the left leg is taken further back to open and stretch through the hip. Place a cushion under the right knee and in the last few weeks under the abdomen as well. This can be altered for your complete comfort. Once you have made all the necessary adjustments to your position and cushions, close your eyes and relax into the pose.

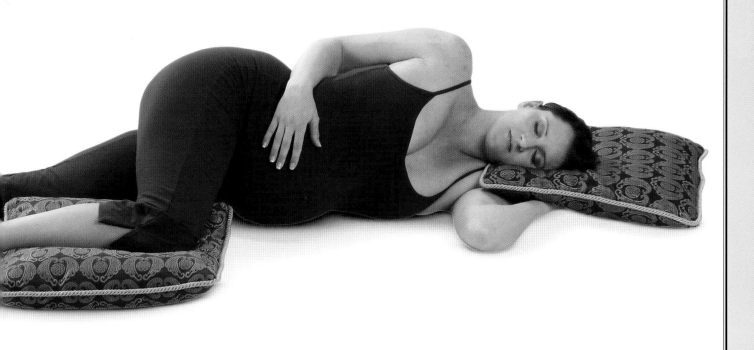

PELVIC ROCKING

Pelvic Rocking can be enjoyed throughout your pregnancy as a gentle way to massage and relax deeply into the pelvic area, especially if you have lower-back pain. When you are on the hands and knees, the weight of the baby is moved away from your body helping to relieve pressure and heaviness. This is very useful if the baby is pressing high under the ribs or causing heavy discomfort in the pelvis. It is often used during labour if your baby is in the posterior position causing back discomfort, or just as a very comfortable way to move through the contractions.

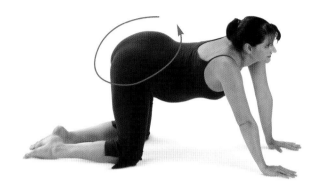

1 Come onto the hands and the knees with the back straight, the knees are hip-distance apart and the hands are under the shoulders. Make big slow circles with the hips to rotate fully into the pelvis, coming far enough forward to feel the weight on the hands and pulling back where the stretch is felt through the whole back. This can be repeated 5 times in one direction and then the other, or as many times as you wish. Resting in the Pose of the Child (see p. 26) follows this exercise very well and both are recommended to use during labour.

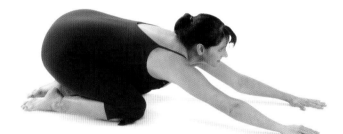

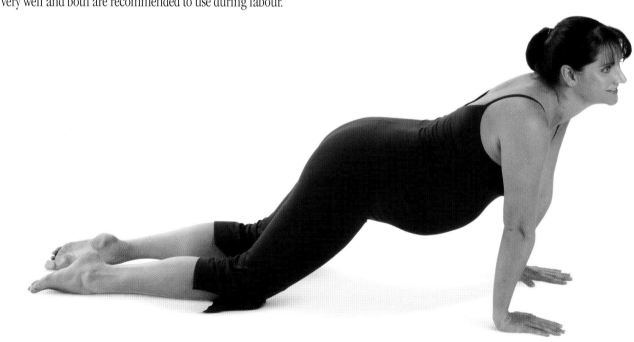

CONTEMPLATION, INNER REFLECTION, MINDFULNESS

Remembering to take a few moments in your day to pause and reflect will encourage a quieter, more peaceful and conscious state of mind where you bring the mind back home to yourself – to contemplate, to meditate and to witness more clearly your inner and outer world. Before you begin your yoga practice and also after you have finished spend some quiet moments alone and at peace with yourself just being there, in the present moment, aware of how your body feels, mindful of the nature of your thoughts and the atmosphere of your mind. Notice the natural breath as it moves gently in and out of the body and feel yourself relaxing and becoming still as you simply observe the breathing and find comfort in that. Feel your baby deep in the womb and spend some quiet time together now, before the birth, resting your mind gently there, with thoughts of love and welcome to your baby. When you put the world on hold for just one or two minutes you create the opportunity and the space to enjoy this brief reflective time, so you can move on through your day with a clear mind, a relaxed body and a sense of calm.

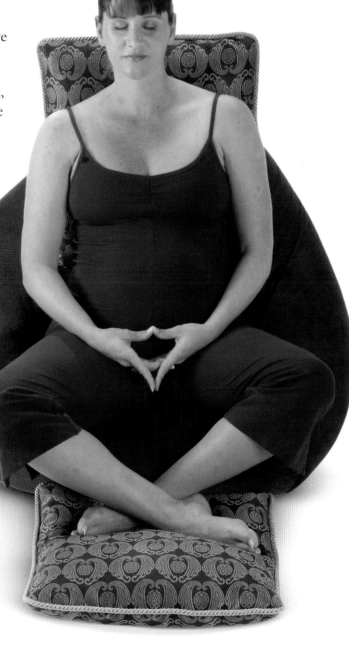

PELVIC FLOOR EXERCISES

The pelvic floor exercises are one of the most important group of exercises that all women should consider doing as regularly as possible, not only during pregnancy and after birth, but throughout adult life too, primarily because they play such an important role in maintaining optimum health and function to the whole pelvic region.

The pelvic floor consists of a complex group of interlocking, overlapping muscles that support the upper body and play an important role in maintaining the health and proper function of the whole pelvic region. They contain the orifices leading to the urethra, the vaginal passage, the womb and the rectum. Under normal circumstances there is a natural pressure on these muscles due to the effects of gravity and because it is quite natural to bear down when emptying the bladder and bowel. During pregnancy the demands are far greater due to increased body weight and blood volume within the pelvic region, resulting in increased pressure on the pelvic floor muscles. It is therefore essential to keep these muscles as firm and strong as possible during pregnancy through regular practice of the pelvic floor exercises but also to ensure that these muscles will continue to be strong not only after the birth but for the rest of your life too.

Even if a woman has never had a vaginal delivery or had children, these exercises need to be practised regularly throughout adult life to prevent problems occurring later on. Although it is usually women who are encouraged to do these exercises they are also highly recommended for men as they can play an important role in maintaining health in the prostate gland and bladder as well as strengthening the muscles that support the lower back and pelvic areas.

WHY SHOULD WE DO PELVIC FLOOR EXERCISES?

When the pelvic floor exercises are practised regularly they will tone and strengthen these important muscles and help prevent a number of problems occurring during pregnancy and after the birth. The problems that can be minimised and often prevented include urinary incontinence which is quite common after giving birth, especially noticeable when you go for a run, cough or sneeze. They are also considered valuable in the prevention and management of haemorrhoids and as an additional treatment if prolapses occur. They help to tone the muscles of the pelvic area and the lower back and should be practised if lower-back weakness occurs. Regular practice will also help you to identify where these muscles are so that you can have more control of them particularly during the second stage of labour.

HOW ARE THEY DONE?

The pelvic floor exercises are very easy to do and can be done anywhere and at any time. As a guideline, simply concentrate on the area from the top of the pubic bone at the front of the body and the corresponding area in the back of the body, or more specifically the parts of the body that would be in contact with the seat of a bicycle or saddle. Concentrate on this area and then lift and tighten the pelvic floor muscles, holding the lift for as long as you can and then relax.

It is important to note that the abdominal muscles are not involved when the pelvic floor exercises are practised and should remain relaxed throughout. Repeat this as many times as you wish, or practise a minimum of between 10 to 30 each day, 10 being better than none at all. For example, do 10 at breakfast, lunch and dinner, which will give you an easy-to-remember, daily routine.

Other variations include counting to five to lift the pelvic floor muscles, hold the lift for five and then relaxing. Alternatively, tighten the pelvic floor muscles while breathing in and relax them while breathing out. Practising daily or as often as you remember will greatly strengthen these muscles and help to avoid unnecessary problems developing now and later in life. To check you are using the pelvic floor muscles correctly, try to stop the flow of urine midstream – it is these muscles that are contracting during this time.

From a traditional yogic perspective these exercises are a combination of two separate practices, one being *moola bandha*, where it is the cervical area in women that is being held and tightened, and *ashwini mudra*, where the anus is tightened. When you become very skilled with these exercises you will be able to do them separately as well as together.

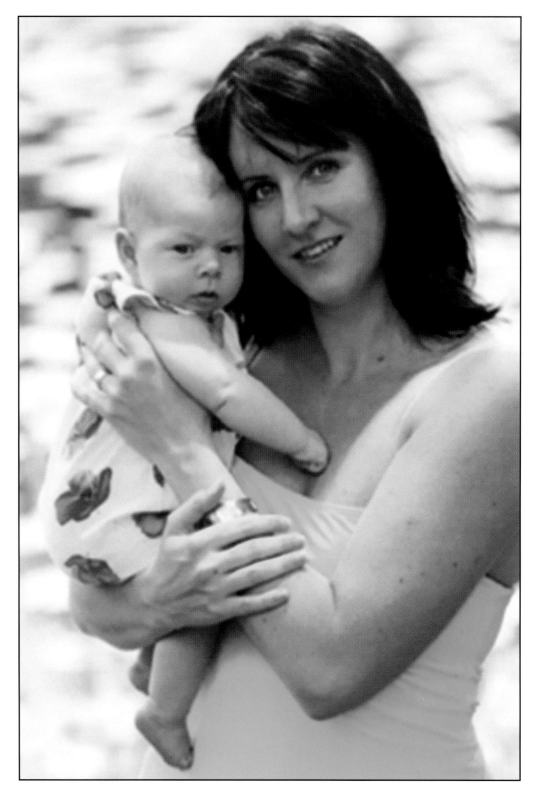

Lisa Newland with her baby Lucia – *photographed by Theresa Jamieson*

CONCLUSION

Pregnancy is a brief and very precious time in your life – it is a unique time where you have the opportunity to nurture and honour yourself as a woman in preparation for becoming a mother. It is a time completely different from any other in your life where you will want to slow down a little and contemplate the many changes that are naturally occurring, not only within your body and your mind but in all aspects of your life as well.

Early in your pregnancy you will find that your needs instinctively change as your energy levels decrease and you will want to rest more as your body adjusts to the changes that are taking place, moment to moment. You might also find that you intuitively withdraw a little from the usual pace of your daily life and find comfort in retreat, becoming more content to simply be and to reflect on the unknowns of this mysterious and challenging new role you are about to embrace – motherhood.

Yoga is about the establishment of a union between the body, the mind and the spirit. Through the gentle practice of yoga you are able to quietly turn your attention inwards and take more intimate care of all your needs during this time – physically, mentally and emotionally and to move through your pregnancy with a sense of grace and ease. Spending time practising the different aspects of yoga and on inner reflection will give you the opportunity to connect with your unborn baby in the womb and to acknowledge the miracle of life and the wonder of being a woman. And because yoga promotes a strong, yet gentle balance within the mind and the body it encourages you to discover from within yourself the invaluable qualities of acceptance and surrender during pregnancy and especially childbirth, and to trust in your own inherent feminine wisdom.

ABOUT THE AUTHOR

THERESA JAMIESON began teaching yoga and meditation in 1980 and specialising in yoga for pregnancy after her first son was born in 1984. She has continued to work with pregnant women, finding that the many different aspects of this gentle form of yoga are a most effective and nurturing way for a woman to maintain excellent physical and emotional health during pregnancy, whilst also being a wonderful way to prepare for becoming a mother. She is a qualified naturopath, herbalist and massage therapist and has studied hypnotherapy and counselling. Theresa uses all these skills in conjunction with yoga and meditation in her work with pregnant women and other people as well. She is the author of *The Complete Book of Yoga and Meditation for Pregnancy* and has a number of audio recordings available. She has a centre in the Gold Coast hinterland where she works and teaches general yoga and yoga for pregnancy, and conducts workshops on preparing for birth.

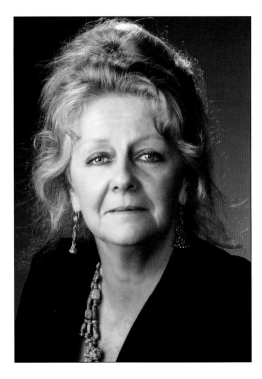

FOR MORE INFORMATION GO TO
www.yoga4pregnancy.com.au

Lisa Newland, who carried out the poses for the book and DVD, was 37 weeks pregnant when the filming was done.

All author's royalties from this book are being donated to Tibetan refugee children in Northern India.